Don't Put *That* in *There*!

Don't Put That in There!

AND 69 OTHER SEX MYTHS DEBUNKED

DR. AARON E. CARROLL AND DR. RACHEL C. VREEMAN

WITHDRAWN

ST. MARTIN'S GRIFFIN ⚞ NEW YORK

DON'T PUT *THAT* IN *THERE!* Copyright © 2014 by Aaron E. Carroll and Rachel C. Vreeman. All rights reserved. Printed in the United States of America. For information, address St. Martin's Press, 175 Fifth Avenue, New York, N.Y. 10010.

www.stmartins.com

Library of Congress Cataloging-in-Publication Data

Carroll, Aaron E.
  Don't put that in there! : and 69 other sex myths debunked / Dr. Aaron E. Carroll and Dr. Rachel C. Vreeman.—First edition.
       pp. cm,
  ISBN 978-1-250-04226-2 (paperback)
  ISBN 978-1-4668-4003-4 (e-book)
  1. Sexual health—Miscellanea.   2. Sex—Miscellanea.   3. Sex (Biology)—Miscellanea.   I. Vreeman, Rachel C.   II. Title.
  RA788.C37 2014
  613.9'5—dc23
                                                              2014008531

St. Martin's Griffin books may be purchased for educational, business, or promotional use. For information on bulk purchases, please contact Macmillan Corporate and Premium Sales Department at 1-800-221-7945, extension 5442, or write specialmarkets@macmillan.com.

First Edition: July 2014

10   9   8   7   6   5   4   3   2   1

Contents

Introduction 1

Part I: Men
Penis Size Matters 7

Batters Up! The Battle of
the 7-Inch Penis. 14

Big Feet, Big Hands, Big . . . ?.........................18

Racial Penis Profiling 22

You Don't Last Long Enough 25

You Shouldn't Have Sex Before
the Big Game..28

Foreskin and Seven Years Ago 31

Your Balls Sag with Age...................................36

Wait for a Whopping Wad...............................39

Start Small, Stay Small 42

Don't Swallow Your Cum! 44

There's Always Semen
When You're Screamin'....................................46

You're Going to Break
That Boner 48

You Are Going to Pump That
Geyser Dry 50

Part II: Women
Wearing a Bra Will Keep Your
Boobs from Sagging 55

Women Don't Really Want Sex 58

Bald Is Best (The Bush Versus
the Brazilian) 62

G-men, G-spots—They Don't Exist!..................67

Women Do Not Squirt
Like Men 72

Blonds Have More Fun....................................77

Nobody Has Pubic Hair
These Days 81

Little Lost Tampon, Where
Did It Go? 85

A Woman Needs Her Clitoris
Stimulated to Have an Orgasm........................88

Buy Our Product for That
Clean, Fresh Feeling! 92

Bigger Breasts
Are Less Sensitive 94

That Hole Does
Nothing for Me 97

Part III: Sex

Oysters, Chocolate, Bananas . . .
Viagra?..101

Don't Put *That* in *There*! 106

It Will Really Turn a
Woman On If You Do
the Laundry 114

Don't Leave Your Socks On!............................117

Lose Weight Fast! Have Sex!..........................119

To Be or Not to Be . . . Pierced 121

Methuselah Had Sex
Ten Times a Day...124

Squeezing Breasts Is All Fun
and Games..127

Get Out of Those Pajamas!.............................129

Can't Buy Me Love 130

Television Makes You
Oversexed..134

It's Only a Matter of Time
Until a Man Cheats...136

There's a Ten-Year Difference
in Sexual Peaks...139

Only Teenagers Come Too Soon......................141

Watching Porn Is a Guy Thing........................144

Men Want It More. Way,
Way More. 147

I Can't Do That . . . It Will
Give Me Hemorrhoids 150

You'll Never Go Gray . . .
Down There..153

Let's Play Back Door, Front
Door, Back Door 155

Married People Don't Play—
with Themselves! 158

Women Are Turned Off by
Sweaty, Stinky Men 160

When in Doubt, Double-Bag It 162

The Stiff Has a Stiff...164

Did She or Didn't She?
Faking It for Beginners. 166

Only Men Have Wet Dreams 168

Masturbation Will Make
You Go Blind..170

Sex Can Give You a Heart
Attack...172

Part IV: Getting Pregnant

You Can't Get Pregnant
During Your Period 177

If a Woman Has an Orgasm,
It Is More Likely She Will
Get Pregnant 179

You Can't Get Pregnant
If It Was a Rape...183

The Pill Will Make You Fat 185

Birth Control Pills Don't Work
as Well If You're on Antibiotics 187

If You Put on the Pounds,
Birth Control Pills Won't Work.......................189

IUDs Are Horrible! 192

Want a Baby Girl? Turn This
Way, Bend That Way. 197

You Can't Get Pregnant If 200

Part V: Sexually Transmitted Infections

You Didn't Get That STD
from Sex...207

But What About Crabs?
I Know You Can Get Those
from the Toilet Seat!...210

Oral Sex Is Totally Safe...................................212

Condoms Will Protect You from
Anything..215

You Don't Need the HPV Vaccine
If You're Not Having Sex 218

The HPV Vaccine Encourages
Girls to Have Sex...221

You Better Not Kiss Anyone
with HIV..224

Anal Sex Will Give You
Cancer 228

References 231

Acknowledgments 257

Index 259

About the Authors 271

Don't Put *That* in *There*!

Introduction

Who do you ask when you have a question about sex? Are there things about sex you've always wondered about, but never dared to bring up with anyone?

Most of us have learned all sorts of things about sex. But, think about where you got your information. You talked about sex with your friends, you learned some basics from your sex ed class, you saw some interesting things on TV or on the Internet, and you figured some things out from experience.

You may have plenty of information about sex, but we would bet that some of it is wrong. People believe all kinds of things about sex that are just not true! And even if you like talking about sex, you might not be as eager to ask questions about whether your ideas about sex are correct.

People believe many myths, half-truths, and outright lies when it comes to sex. When we wrote our first myth-busting book, *Don't Swallow Your Gum!* we included a whole section on myths about sex and getting pregnant. They were hugely popular. When we wrote *Don't Cross Your Eyes . . . ,* we added some more myths in this vein. Once again, the sex myths seemed to be the ones people wanted to talk about most.

After all, who doesn't love talking about sex?

Well . . . believe it or not, it was not our dream to become sex experts! Sex is not all we want to talk about.

Aaron's favorite story about writing our first myth-busting

book is how much he teased Rachel over her inability to defend whether "cum" should or should not be spelled with a "u." Ask her. Watch her blush.

Aaron has three kids who are still pretty young, and he has had a hard time deflecting conversations about this book from them. His daughter, age seven at the time of writing this, seems to be on to him, and is constantly pressuring him for more information about the book.

Nonetheless, as pediatricians, part of our job is to teach adolescents about sex. As researchers, our job is to help figure out the science about what works and what doesn't work to keep people healthy. And as professional myth-debunkers, we can't let you believe things about sex and your body that just are not true.

So, we overcame our inhibitions to shine some light (and evidence) on the most popular and prevalent sex myths around. For those of you who are new to these books, here's how it all works:

One of the skills necessary to our job as health services researchers is to understand health research and translate what it means for the general public. So for each of these myths, we scoured the world's medical literature, looking for scientific studies to prove the idea true or false. You'd be shocked at how often real research has been done on these topics. We bring the science to you, explain what it means, and—more often than not—detail why these myths are or aren't true.

When you read this book, it's important that you remember we do not just want to give you our opinions. We're showing you, through data, why we think an idea is a myth. We won't just tell you that myths aren't real; we'll show you why.

This is the book that will answer all those crazy questions you have had about sex. Plus, if you read it, you're pretty much guaranteed to be the life of the party. Our friends love just hearing the chapter titles in this book. Imagine how popular you'll be when you become the sexpert who can discuss them at length.

Some of the myths in this book are lighthearted fun. Others are deadly serious. We apply the same research and scrutiny to all of them. If we can't find evidence, we'll say so. But more often than not, science exists to tell us whether that sex idea is true or myth. When there is science, we should use it. Get ready for all of the sex science.

Happy myth-busting!

Part One

MEN

Penis Size Matters

One of our friends debunks the myth this way: "It's not the size of the wave, but the motion of the ocean." There are a lot of different ways to phrase this, but it comes down to one important question: Does it matter how big the guy's penis is? We will start by looking at whether penis size matters to men who have sex with women, then whether it matters to the women themselves, and then whether it matters to men who have sex with men.

If you ask your friends, you might hear all kinds of answers to this question. Some claim that size does not matter at all as long as the man knows how to use their penis well. Others swear that the best sex of their lives was with a particularly well-endowed partner. And some will say that sex with an exceptionally large penis was not enjoyable, and even painful. Both popular opinion and surveys suggest that men are very concerned about the question of how big they are and how the size of their penis compares to other men's penises.

Scientists have looked at the influence of penis size on all sorts of things—from height and body fat to sexual satisfaction and the risk of having various infections. The studies tell us that penis size does matter, but not necessarily in the ways that you might think.

A huge Internet survey of more than 50,000 heterosexual men and women investigated penis size and satisfaction. In this survey, most men reported that they had an average-sized penis (66 percent), while 22 percent said their penis was large and 12 percent rated it as small. No actual penis sizes were measured, so this study relied only on what these men said about themselves. (Remember, they might not have the right idea about what an average penis size really is!) About half of the men (55 percent) were satisfied with their penis size, but 45 percent wanted to have a larger penis and 0.2 percent wanted to be smaller. In contrast, 85 percent of women reported being satisfied with their partner's penis size. This suggests that size is less important to women, or that they are more likely to be satisfied with their partner's penis size, than he is with his own size.

In this study, reporting that you had a big penis was linked to other body traits that are generally thought to be good. The self-reported penis size correlated positively with being taller and with having less body fat. The men reporting having larger penises also reported being more attractive. While some people might call that good luck or good genes—whatever it is that makes you both well-endowed and handsome—this finding could also reflect very confident individuals who think that everything about themselves is great, from how handsome they are to how big their penis is. This is one of those unexpected ways in which penis size might matter. How you see your penis might be correlated with how you see the rest of you.

Other studies have looked at how penis size, body shape, and height might be related to each other. Scientists have wondered whether evolution pushed these traits together because women might have considered all of them when they were considering their mating options. An evolutionary force might be at play if women were making their decisions about who to mate with based on whom they found the most attractive. If women found penis size very attractive, then women might be more likely to pick men with bigger penises, and then humans might be pushed toward having bigger and bigger penises.

Along these lines, scientists wanted to assess how much penis size plays into women's ideas about who is attractive. To do this, they set up studies where women evaluate life-sized digital pictures of men of various proportions. It turns out that penis size, body shape, and height are all significant factors in who women think are hot. Increasing penis size in these digital men did increase how often women thought they were attractive, but the effect got smaller and smaller past a certain point. Penis size actually had a stronger effect on attractiveness in taller men than in shorter men, and the same was true for men with a more masculine body shape (which is defined as having wider shoulders and narrower hips). This means that increasing the size of the penis on a taller man got them a higher rating of attractiveness than increasing the size of the penis by the same amount for a shorter man. It turns out that height and penis size matter about the same in these judgments of attractiveness. Larger penis size and taller height had almost the exact same influence on a woman's rating of the man as attractive.

Of course, just because penis size may factor into a woman's judgment of how attractive someone looks does not mean that this will influence their decisions about their partners. After all, 85 percent of the women in that big survey did say they were satisfied with their partner's penis size. Plus, an important question remains: Does penis size actually influence sexual pleasure?

One study does suggest that penis size may make a difference for women's orgasms. A study of 323 women investigated how often they had penile-vaginal intercourse (that means sex with a penis in the vagina), vaginal orgasms, and clitoral orgasms. (To read more about the many ways women can have orgasms, see the fun chapters on whether a woman needs her clitoris stimulated to have an orgasm and whether women have orgasms through anal sex!) The study's whole goal was to figure out whether having sex with someone with a longer penis made you more likely to have a vaginal orgasm. According to this study, it kind of does!

It turns out that women who prefer deeper penis stimulation are more likely to have vaginal orgasms. This was not a study that could show cause and effect. The link between long penises, deep stimulation, and vaginal orgasms could mean that a longer penis gives you more vaginal orgasms, but it also could simply mean that women who say they prefer longer penises are more likely to have vaginal orgasms. It does not mean that the longer penis is more likely to cause a vaginal orgasm, but that the women who are having those vaginal orgasms think that the longer penis might be a good thing. In this study, these women also placed less importance on non-coital sex (sex that did not involve the penis being inside the vagina). Still, this suggests that there might be a subset of women for whom penis length makes a difference in their sexual experience.

Despite this limited evidence that size might affect some

women's experiences, having the right moves might make up for any perceived deficiencies. Sex therapists and specialists can teach you something called "Coital Alignment Technique," which has been evaluated in a series of controlled studies. In these studies, certain positions or "ineffective" intercourse techniques are shown to cause sexual problems like women not being able to have orgasms during penile-vaginal intercourse or premature ejaculation. However, using the "Coital Alignment Technique" increases the odds of the woman having an orgasm during penile-vaginal intercourse. (In other words, these moves alone could lead to vaginal orgasms, regardless of the penis size.)

Find yourself wondering just what this "Coital Alignment Technique" is? It sounds a little complicated, but here is what it entails: A man lies right on top of a woman, but moves himself far enough up along the woman's body that his erection is actually pointing down, so that the top side of the penis presses against the clitoris. To thrust deeper inside, the man actually moves his body down compared to the woman, and then moves back up as he withdraws. The man and woman are supposed to focus on the movement of their pelvises and not on support or movement using their arms or legs.

Good luck with that!

Here's another interesting question: Does penis size matter when it comes to men who have sex with men?

There is not much scientific literature describing what penis size means among men who have sex with men, but one study surveying 1,065 men who have sex with men did evaluate how the men's perception of their penises influenced other characteristics of their sexual health.

In this group, 7.1 percent reported their penis size was "below average," 56.0 percent described it as "average," and 36.9 percent called their penis size "above average." Among the entire group of men, reported penis size did not seem to make any difference for the number of sex partners, frequency of sex, condom use, or likelihood of having HIV or other sexually transmitted infections including gonorrhea, chlamydia, syphilis, urinary tract infections, or hepatitis.

In contrast, men who reported an "above average" penis size were statistically more likely to be satisfied with their penis size and less likely to lie about its size. They were also more likely to report two things that no one wants to have—genital warts and herpes. The correlation between having a larger penis and having more genital warts or herpes infections is interesting because both of these infections are caused by viruses that can be passed from one person to another if any affected part of the penis or the skin around it isn't covered by a condom. This connection made the authors of the study wonder whether the larger penis size meant these men had more issues with condoms slipping or breaking, both of which could leave contagious skin exposed and increase the chance of infections.

Among men who have sex with men, their perceived penis size might also impact the sexual position they assume during sex, as well as their psychosocial adjustment. In this study, men who reported having "below average"-sized penises were significantly more likely to identify themselves as "bottoms," meaning that they were the ones on the receiving end of anal sex. In contrast, the men who said they had "above average"-sized penises were significantly more likely to call themselves "tops," meaning that they were the ones doing the insertion during anal intercourse. In addition, the men who rated their penis size as "below average" also scored significantly worse on three different measures of psychosocial adjustment. All of these findings suggest that one's perception of one's penis size among the group of men who have sex with men might play a significant role in certain sexual behaviors and psychosocial adjustment.

What do all of these studies suggest about penis size? Does penis size matter? The take-home message is that penis size may make a difference for some things (like how you feel about yourself and whether you lie about your penis), but it does not necessarily affect your partner's satisfaction with you.

Batters Up! The Battle of the 7-Inch Penis.

You cannot talk about sex for too long without getting into a discussion about penis size. A huge amount of worry, energy, speculation, and wonder seems to be devoted to whether or not a penis "measures up." From men claiming to be well-endowed, to those secretly worrying that there is just not something large enough in their pants, to endless junk e-mails about how to enlarge your penis, the size of the male member gets a lot of press.

Whether penis size matters at all is another question (keep reading for that chapter!), but many people do not even know how their penis (or another penis that they care about) compares in size to the world's penis population. Is your penis below average in size? Above average? You would be surprised at how few people can answer this question correctly.

To make a judgment on how a penis measures up, you have to think about two things: First is the size of the average penis. And, second, are you talking about a flaccid penis or an erect penis? An erection brings about a dramatic size change in penis size as it fills with blood.

Do you have your rulers ready? Figuring out the size of the average penis is more of a challenge than you might think. It is hard to get an accurate picture of penis size when you ask men to report their own measurements. Perhaps this surprises no one, but men tend to exaggerate the length of their penises, and they don't take the most exact measurements of their own members. Still, we can get some idea of average penis size when we get lots and lots of men to measure their penises.

A large Internet survey that collected penis size and other information from 2,545 men found that the average length of the erect penis was 6.4 inches (with a standard deviation of 1.2 inches). These averages were based on men's own measurements of their erect penises.

In another study done by Indiana University researchers at The Kinsey Institute, the average erect penis size among 1,661 American men was 5.6 inches. Interestingly enough, in this study, the average size was different based on how the man got the erection. The men who had received oral sex and then measured their erection reported larger sizes than the men who got their erection from self-masturbation or hand stimulation by a partner. You can't really figure out why these differences exist from this type of study. It's possible that oral sex gives you a larger erection, but it's also possible that men with larger erect penises are more likely to get oral sex.

Based on these surveys, 7 inches should not be your benchmark for normal. In studies where men themselves report the size of their member, the average erect penis size is 5.6 to 6.4 inches. Not 7 inches. When most people talk about "average," they mean the size that is the most common. The most common measurement was more along the lines of 6 inches for an erect penis—and that still may have been an overestimation. Just because 6 inches was the most common does not mean that something else is "not normal." It's also completely normal to have penises that are smaller or larger than that.

In case you want to compare other penis measurements, in the largest survey, the average length of the flaccid, or soft, penis was 3.4 inches, the average circumference of the erect penis was 5 inches, and the average length of the head of the penis was 1.6 inches. In the study of 1,661 American men, the average circumference of the erect penis was 4.8 inches.

These surveys give us some idea of what the average penis length may be, but we still have the problem of men reporting that their members are a bit longer than they really are. To get the most accurate measures of the male member, it works best to have specialists take the measurements, and so we look to studies with measurements done by urologists.

The studies by the specialists do not include as many men, but they should give us more scientific estimates of what is average. While urologists agree that the erect penile length is the most physiologically accurate measurement, they usually use "stretched penile length" for their studies. Rather than requiring the men in the study to get an erection, the doctors doing these studies take a soft penis, stretch it out, and measure the length with a measuring tape. This stretched length is considered a good substitute for measuring the erect penis.

We found fifteen studies where objective scientists measured the stretched penile length for a group of men. In these studies, the average penile lengths found among the men ranged quite a bit, from 3.5 inches to 6.6 inches. Most of the studies (nine of fifteen) had averages in the range of 4.7 to 5.1

inches. You will note that these averages are at least an inch shorter than the measurements that men reported for themselves in the Internet survey, and the average measurements all remain less than 7 inches. In fact, the average seemed to be much closer to 5 inches.

You can put your rulers away now.

Big Feet, Big Hands, Big . . . ?

We started our very first book of medical myths—*Don't Swallow Your Gum! Myths, Half-Truths, and Outright Lies About Your Body and Health*—debunking the myth that men with big feet have big penises. No book discussing sex myths would be complete without a discussion of whether you can predict who is well-endowed. In our years of experience talking about medical myths at cocktail parties or dinners, we almost always get asked about this one. Of course, that might just be because people like to see whether Rachel blushes when she talks about penis size. (She usually does.)

Many people think that you can size up what a man's penis is going to be like by sneaking a peek at other parts of him. Large feet, hands, and noses are all rumored to tell you that the appendage in a man's pants is also going to be large. And men with small hands or feet will tell you that they hate how everyone jumps to conclusions that they will be smaller in size elsewhere.

Interestingly enough, the connection between big feet and big penises has some roots in science. A particular gene called the Hox gene plays a role in the development of the toes and fingers, as well as the penis and clitoris. If the same gene controls the growth of toes, fingers, and penises, then it might make all of them grow big (or not).

However, as scientific as it sounds to speculate that control by the same gene leads to the simultaneous growth of extra-large feet and extra-large penises, we don't think that most people make the leap to connect penis size with foot size because they are experts in genetics. It is much more likely that this myth comes from the human tendency to identify patterns. We like to have explanations for things we see, and we like to group similar things together (like big feet and big penises). Of course, an intense interest in the size of an organ that has not yet been seen or experienced is also a good motivator for coming up with a way to predict its size. Inquiring minds want to know!

Even though the same genes play a role in the growth of penises, hands, and feet, there is no good evidence that men with big feet have bigger penises. Scientific studies of penis size produce somewhat mixed results, but they lean in favor of there being no connection.

As you might recall, some measurements of the penis are more accurate than others. If you have a penis, you are not the best person to measure it. The most-trustworthy way to measure the penis is to have someone else do it, ideally an objective researcher who follows the same measurement technique for measuring every penis. You might call them professional penis pullers, since the most accurate way to measure the penis is to take a soft penis, stretch it out to its full length, and then measure it, as we describe in the chapter on whether the average penis size is really 7 inches.

One study of 63 men in Canada looking at stretched penis length and shoe size did find a weak, but statistically significant relationship between the length of the penis and shoe size, as well as a correlation between penis length and height. This study did not actually measure the men's feet, though, but relied on their reported shoe size. In contrast, a slightly larger study that looked at stretched penile length and shoe size for 104 men found no correlation between the length of the penis and the size of the shoe. These are pretty mixed results; one says that the two are weakly connected to each other, and the other says that they are not. Plus, they are both small studies. We do not have great science on this one.

Studies where men measure and report their own penis lengths are not considered to have the most accurate measurements since they might exaggerate. Nonetheless, less-than-ideal studies can still give us a general idea about what is true. In this case, while the Internet survey where lots of men measured their own penises might not be as accurate, it could be a tiebreaker for the other two studies.

"The Definitive Penis Size Survey," in which 3,100 men reported information about the sizes of their penis and their other characteristics, found no relationship between shoe size and erect penis size. Again, we have to remember that this study used only men's own measurements. Furthermore, it is not the strongest science since "The Definitive Penis Size Survey" was never reviewed by other experts or published in a scientific journal. However, the survey seems to have been reasonably well done, and the results do back up the findings that the scientific studies showed either no connection or a weak connection.

We could not find any studies evaluating whether the size of the hands or of the nose are connected to penis size. Since the combined evidence suggests foot size and penis size are not linked, there's no reason to believe that hand size or nose size or any other body part would predict penis size.

Our conclusion? You can look at a guy's feet all you want, but it is only going to give you an idea about his taste in shoes. The size of his feet (or hands, or nose) will not give you a good idea of how the rest of him measures up.

Racial Penis Profiling

There are quite a number of racial stereotypes built into this myth, and we have to say from the beginning that it is difficult to wade through the studies without getting trapped in controversies about race and about how people are viewed. However, we get a lot of questions about whether penis size really is different among one group compared to another. When it comes to the myths, one most often hears that black men have the largest penises, Asian men have the smallest penises, and everyone else lands somewhere in between.

The best answer is that we don't know. There hasn't been a systematic and objective evaluation of penis size that compares penis sizes across various racial or ethnic populations. By systematic, we mean that the study is designed to sample men from various ethnic groups according to good scientific methods. Moreover, the existing studies that compare penis size and ethnicity do not use the most accurate type of penis measurements. Rather than using an objective observer or a scientist who can document the stretched penile length, the existing work relies on Internet surveys in which men report how long their penis is. As we mentioned previously, when men are taking their own measurements, the measurements are not very accurate.

One study that has gotten a lot of press looks at reports of penis lengths from across 113 countries. This report made the media go crazy with a list ranking men's average penis size by country. The Democratic Republic of Congo was at the top of the list for average penis size, followed by Ecuador, Ghana, and Columbia. Several northeast Asian countries were at the bottom of the list. Does this mean the stereotypes are true?

No! While the research, conducted by a psychologist named Richard Lynn, seems good at first glance, it suffers from a number of problems. It just wasn't a high-quality study to answer the question of whether penis size is tied to ethnicity. It wasn't designed to measure penis size objectively, or to estimate penis sizes in various parts of the world. Instead, it relied on reports of penis size from Internet-based surveys or collected from Web sites. These aren't the most accurate data on penis length. Without good science to support this claim, we remain highly skeptical. We need a study that is designed to give us good answers, or else we can't believe the results.

It is also relevant to know that Dr. Lynn is a psychologist who is known for *very* controversial views on race and intelligence, and who makes arguments for things like selecting out embryos to increase the intelligence of a population. What most of the media articles did not report is that his recent paper describing how penis size might vary from one country to another is intended to examine how penis size differences would support a particular evolutionary theory about how different races evolve in different ways, claiming that some races prioritize reproduction, while others prioritize parenting. The conclusions of this study are intended to support the very controversial (and many would say racist) idea of another researcher, J. Philippe Rushton, who claimed that the populations that "left Africa" developed in a way that required "larger brains, more family stability, and a longer life," balanced by "lower levels of sex hormones" and "less sexual activity" (and, therefore, smaller penises). Dr. Rushton directed an organization called the Pioneer Fund, and Dr. Lynn sits on its board of directors. This organization is routinely accused of racism, and even of white supremacism, because it funds a lot of research on racial differences in IQ.

This all means that the paper describing these differences in penis size from one country to another may be biased to fit the author's particular viewpoint. Many scientists have raised concerns about Dr. Lynn's claims. We especially worry that you cannot trust his study's findings, since the methodology wasn't very good to begin with.

Given all of these concerns, we would strongly caution against jumping to conclusions about whether penis size really does vary with ethnicity or what part of the world you're from. If we're going to answer this question, we need much better science.

You Don't Last Long Enough

A lot of men worry that they ejaculate too quickly. This can cause them significant concern, and it can cause distress for their partners as well, if either party would like for the man to last longer.

"Premature ejaculation" is the official term for ejaculating too quickly. You may be surprised to learn that the definition of "too quickly" is not entirely clear. The official word on the topic is that premature ejaculation is an orgasm that happens before the penis is inserted in the vagina, or within about one minute of having the penis in the vagina. The guidelines on premature ejaculation only look at premature ejaculation in intravaginal intercourse (meaning sex with a penis inside a vagina), so what we describe next does not apply to other sexual behaviors, or to men having sex with men.

You have to meet three criteria to get diagnosed with premature ejaculation: 1) you have a short time before you ejaculate (you always or nearly always have an orgasm before or within a minute of penetrating the vagina), 2) you do not feel able to control the timing of your ejaculation once you are inside the vagina, and 3) you are distressed or bothered by this. If you have your orgasm between 1 and 1.5 minutes after you enter the vagina and meet these other criteria, you have "probable" premature ejaculation.

According to the studies compiled by the International Society for Sexual Medicine's official committee on premature ejaculation, somewhere between 22 and 30 percent of men report premature ejaculation when you don't put a time limit on the concern. When you specify a time parameter of less than 1 minute, only 1 to 3 percent meet the criteria for having a problem.

If less than 1 minute is considered a problem for your sexual health, then what is the normal time for a man to last once his penis enters the vagina? It may still be shorter than you would think.

In a study of 500 European and American men, the average man's "intravaginal ejaculation latency time" (i.e., how long between entering the vagina and orgasm) was 5.4 minutes. The men were clocked with a stopwatch in the course of a month of having sex with their regular female partners. All of the men were in stable relationships during the four weeks of the study. The men's time before ejaculating did vary dramatically; the shortest recorded time was 0.55 minutes and the longest was 44.1 minutes. You may be especially surprised to learn that younger men in this study were actually able to last longer. The median time to ejaculation was 6.5 minutes for those ages eighteen to thirty, whereas it went down to 5.4 minutes for those thirty-one to fifty years old and then 4.3 minutes for those over fifty-one years. That's a statistically significant difference among the age groups.

Do you think that a condom might make you last longer? In this study, using a condom made no difference for how long the men lasted. It also did not matter whether they were circumcised or not circumcised. For reasons that could not be explained, men in Turkey had significantly shorter times before ejaculation compared to all of the other countries, but this might have had to do with the small numbers of men from each of the countries involved.

This was a relatively small study, and probably applies best to men in similar situations—those in a stable sexual relationship lasting for at least six months and where sex occurs at least once a week. Using a stopwatch to figure out how long the men lasted may have some drawbacks as well. (A word of advice: A stopwatch in the bedroom may not be the most fun toy to introduce.) However, using a stopwatch is considered the best way to measure timing accurately in the course of a usual sexual event.

Now that you have a better idea about what's normal, let's talk a little more about what you can do if you really do have premature ejaculation. Multiple studies tell us that it has negative effects on both of the people involved, including reports of lower self-esteem and more anxiety for men, and less sexual satisfaction for women. Both partners report that premature ejaculation makes their quality of life worse.

Despite all of this doom and gloom, you can change this. There are quite a number of things that can be done for premature ejaculation. First of all, premature ejaculation sometimes occurs because of other medical problems. It is important to have a doctor assess whether you have such problems, and what might be done about them. Second, there are lots of solutions to this issue. There are medicines that treat premature ejaculation effectively, there are therapies and strategies that help men learn to control their ejaculation more, and there are ways that your partner can help you. If you have this issue, you should ask your doctor about it. While it may seem embarrassing to ask, your doctor can help you figure out how to improve your sexual experiences. That should be well worth a little embarrassment!

You Shouldn't Have Sex Before the Big Game

Competitive athletes will consider almost anything to boost their performances. You hear about them following superstitious rituals, sticking to rigid diet plans, and even taking performance-enhancing drugs. Many athletes are told that they should not have sex the night before a big game or competition. They are even warned against masturbating. Abstaining is supposed to help your performance. Athletes who talk about plans to have one-night stands during the Olympics, or even to stay with their spouses before a big game, are regarded with horror—not because of their moral decisions, but because they might not perform as well.

All sorts of reasons are given as to why you want to abstain from sex before a game. People are afraid that having sex might hurt your performance because you will have less strength, less concentration, or not enough testosterone. Instead of using up their energy in the bedroom, the sexually frustrated athlete can channel all of their strength and focus into an aggressive, strong performance on the track or playing field.

The science of what happens in the body during and after sex suggests that these concerns about sex and sports are just not true. In fact, you might actually perform better if you have sex!

Drs. McGlone and Shrier of McGill University conducted a search for all of the scientific studies that would answer the question of whether or not you should have sex the night before a competition. They only found three scientific studies that actually tested this question, but they found no evidence in these studies that sex would decrease your performance.

First of all, you are unlikely to wear yourself out. While the body does use up some energy when having sex, the average sexual encounter does not last long enough or involve enough exertion to change your athletic performance. Estimates of how many calories are used up during sex range from 25 to 125, but that is not a lot of energy—especially for an athlete! Sex is only considered a mild to moderate intensity activity, and the average sexual encounter only lasts around five minutes. No one has any problem with an athlete walking up one or two flights of stairs before a big game, and that is considered equal to the average sexual encounter.

Now, if you are having exceptionally long and vigorous sex, especially if it involves staying up all night, this might be another story. Exhaustion can certainly affect athletic performance, even if "usual" sex would not.

What about that competitive, testosterone-driven aggression? Will sexual frustration boost your testosterone or save up your testosterone for the big game? In one study, men who had sex the night before a sporting event actually had higher testosterone levels the next day than those who had not had sex. This is a good thing for many sports, because higher testosterone is generally associated with more aggression and more strength. Sex has also been shown to have no impact on leg muscle strength, grip strength, reaction time, or flexibility.

On the other hand, you cannot discount how sex impacts

one very important part of your body—your brain. When it comes to sex, the brain is just as important as other parts of the body. The same is true in sports. Any given individual might have good psychological or emotional reasons why they should or should not have sex before a big competition. If the pursuit of a partner or actually having sex distracts you or hurts your mental focus, then sex might not be good for you before an important athletic event. The psychological impact could be a problem even if the physiological impact should not be one.

In contrast, if you sleep or relax better after sex or if you are a person who performs better when you have some sort of sexual excitement going on, then sex might be exactly what you need before your big competition. Athletes often strive for a balanced state of mind where they are well-rested, alert, and focused, but with just enough anxiety or fear to keep them sharp. For some, sex helps with this state of mind; while for others, maybe it ruins it.

Foreskin and Seven Years Ago . . .

Foreskins, what are they good for?

For such a small part of the body, the foreskin is quite a controversial piece of tissue. For thousands of years, the decision to circumcise or not circumcise the penis was associated with the rules and traditions of certain religions. Wars have been fought over these religious traditions—wars over the foreskin.

While not as horrific as the historical clashes, the battles over the foreskin continue today. You can find anti-circumcision advocates protesting with giant signs about how male circumcision reduces sexual pleasure and constitutes a form of torture.

Whether or not men are circumcised varies dramatically based on where you live. Around the globe, about one-third of males are circumcised, for reasons that vary from religious traditions to medical needs to cultural preference. Currently, baby boys are often circumcised in places like the United States, Canada, Australia, much of the Middle East, and West Africa. Circumcision of male infants is relatively uncommon currently in Europe, East and Southern Africa, and other parts of the world. In some of these places, boys are circumcised later in life; in other parts of the world most men are never circumcised.

In recent years, scientists have made some important new discoveries about the foreskin. One of these discoveries is that male circumcision actually protects against several diseases. Men who have been circumcised are less likely to have urinary tract infections, herpes, syphilis, chancroid, and invasive cancer of the penis. Perhaps the most important discovery along these lines is that being circumcised protects you against HIV. Men who have been circumcised are actually 50 to 60 percent less likely to get HIV. When it comes to preventing HIV, male circumcision seems to be a huge help. Since lots and lots of things do not work to prevent HIV, figuring out that something *does* work is a big deal.

Scientists first got the idea that circumcision might decrease the chance of getting infected with HIV by looking at large databases of men over time, and whether or not they were getting infected with HIV, and then comparing this information to characteristics like being circumcised. This is reasonable science when you have lots and lots of people involved (which these studies did), but now the research has gotten even better. Male circumcision has been studied in very large trials, where adult men are actually randomized to either get circumcised or to not get circumcised. Randomized controlled trials are usually the best type of scientific evidence for proving causality. The results of these trials show that the circumcised men are significantly less likely to get infected with HIV.

Male circumcision also seems to prevent certain infections for women. In particular, two sexually transmitted infections, *Trichomonas* and bacterial vaginosis are less common in women whose partners have undergone circumcision.

These might seem like good reasons to promote circumcision, but there are also a lot of reasons why people are not in favor of circumcision. Like any surgical procedure, there is a risk of bleeding, developing an infection, cutting the wrong thing, or developing a hematoma, or collection of blood. These risks are very low for babies (0.2 to 0.4 percent), but can happen. There seems to be greater risk for complications when you circumcise an adolescent or adult man, but there are not a lot of data on how often problems happen. Whether or not the provider is experienced, whether the procedure happens in a clinical setting, what tools are used, and what kind of follow-up is available, all might contribute to the safety of circumcision.

One of the biggest arguments against male circumcision has been that it decreases the sensation of the penis. This seems to be the reason for most of the protests. There is clear evidence that the foreskin itself is sensitive; it has thousands of nerve endings, and these would be lost when the foreskin is removed. Some small studies have suggested that circumcised men report less sensitivity of the penis, and more problems with erections and ejaculation. There is also a lot of expert theory to support this idea based on what happens to the tissue when you circumcise a man. When you remove the foreskin, the glans or head of the penis is left exposed, which changes the tissue that covers it, making it a drier tissue that might also be less sensitive.

For a long time, this theory and these smaller studies seemed like the best evidence we were going to have on the topic. And yet, we had a big problem with those studies comparing circumcised and uncircumcised men because most of these men grew up with their circumcised or uncircumcised penises and could not really weigh in on the difference that circumcision makes for an adult. They had not experienced it both ways. In the few studies that measured the actual sensitivity of the penis, there did not seem to be a difference. No one thought there would be a day when it was okay to do a study that would randomly assign men to either get circumcised or not get circumcised.

But that all changed when scientists began to question whether circumcision prevented HIV. Suddenly, they needed to answer this important question, and it made sense to get that answer using the best science possible. Scientists then conducted studies involving thousands and thousands of men in Kenya who were randomized to either get circumcised or not get circumcised. (Yes, the men signed up voluntarily to be in the study, so they knew that they were going to be put randomly into one of these groups to either go under the knife or not, and they were okay with that.)

These large, randomized, controlled studies actually gave us very good evidence about the impact of circumcision on men's sexual satisfaction and the sensitivity of their penises. These studies do not show any problems with the penis becoming less sensitive after circumcision or any problems with the men reaching orgasm. In fact, the opposite seems to be true. Overall, the circumcised men actually report that their penises are more sensitive, and that they have an easier time reaching orgasm. These large studies suggest that male circumcision does not hurt men's sexual function at all.

Once you take off a foreskin, it is awfully difficult to put something back on! Because this is such an important question to answer up front, researchers have done an extensive search, called a systematic review, where they collected all of the available studies on the topic, and combined them together into a meta-analysis. When they put ten studies together, combining findings from almost 20,000 men, they did not see any differences between circumcised and uncircumcised men in terms of sexual desire, pain during sex, premature ejaculation, problems with erections, or problems with orgasms. We have a very good answer to the question of whether circumcision creates sexual problems for men.

While the foreskin is certainly a sensitive part of the male anatomy, there can be some benefits to removing it in terms of preventing infections, particularly HIV. The bulk of the existing evidence suggests that circumcision does not hurt a man's sexual experience. These benefits should be considered when one weighs decisions about whether or not circumcision should occur.

Your Balls Sag with Age

A man's scrotum and testicles are an amazingly well-regulated set of equipment. The testicles (aka, testes) are supposed to come down out of the body by the time a baby boy is born, or shortly thereafter. Once the testicles are down, the body does its best to keep the testicles at just the right temperature—not too hot or too cold. The body wants to make sure that the testicles can produce sperm at maximum capacity, and this works best when the temperature is just right.

Testicles will start to grow in size when boys first begin to enter puberty, usually around the age of ten to thirteen years. The sac around them will also start to grow in size, to darken, to hang lower, and to grow hair.

Where exactly the testicles hang is actually a very interesting process. To keep the testes at the right temperature, the skin of the scrotal sac has a layer of muscle that is very sensitive to temperature, touch, and stress. When conditions are warm, the muscles lining the scrotal sac relax, and the testes hang lower down from the body where they can stay cool enough. When conditions are cold, these muscles contract, and everything is held tighter and closer to the body. For some men, these muscles also contract during sex or during times of emotional stress.

Some men actually consider it very desirable to have low-hanging balls. In fact, there is an entire practice dedicated to trying to expand the skin of the scrotal sac to get your testicles to hang lower. For some, this is also considered a very sexually enjoyable practice. Men will even use weights or "ball stretchers" to try to get their scrotum to stretch out. (Photos are not for those faint of heart—or sensitive of scrotum!) Challenges with this practice include dealing with the pain, knowing what to wear with low-hanging balls, and not having your testicles hang in the toilet water when you are trying to go to the bathroom. Despite our mentioning the practice in this book, ball stretching is not physician recommended!

Even if you are not trying to stretch out your scrotum, many people have heard that men will become "low hangers" as they age. They expect a decrease in the strength of those scrotal sac muscles with age and a sagging of the balls to go along with it. Earlobes, breasts, balls—all of these body parts are expected to droop with age.

But, does this really happen? Do a man's balls start to sag with age?

The male reproductive tract definitely goes through a number of changes with age. While the cells in the testicles that make sperm are formed continually, they start to produce fewer sperm, slower sperm, and sperm that are less able to fertilize an egg. Older men's sperm are also more likely to have genetic abnormalities. Very old men can still get a woman pregnant under the right conditions, but it is much less likely than when they are younger because of these issues with sperm production.

The components of the testicles also start to change and wear out with age. The tiny tubes where sperm are produced start to degenerate, as do the other structures within the testicles. Overall, testicles also become smaller. Smaller testicles may seem like they are hanging lower, because the sac itself is just a bit emptier. This might create an illusion of extra droopiness.

There are no real studies on the measurements of where testicles hang over time. It is clear that the biggest change in where the balls hang happens when boys enter puberty and they have that significant increase in the size of the testicles and of the scrotal sac. After that, experts say that the changes are pretty minimal. There might be some weakening of the skin of the scrotal sac, but the smooth muscle that controls the movement of the scrotal sac up and down continues to function for a man's entire life. And that kind of muscle—smooth muscle—is unlikely to sag very much.

Wait for a Whopping Wad

A lot of guys have heard that they will have a lot more ejaculate if it has been a long time since they last came. We have no idea why people seem obsessed with the volume of a man's ejaculate, but obsessed they are. You can read any number of stories on things that increase or decrease the amount of semen that a man will produce when he orgasms.

While the general population seems concerned with the volume of ejaculation, scientists are much more concerned with the actual content of it (i.e., sperm). That's because sperm are what's involved in reproduction, and that's what most doctors and researchers really care about. Nonetheless, we found lots of information in the medical literature about how just much ejaculate comes out when a man comes.

For instance, in 1975, a group of researchers gathered 1,300 men who had fathered at least two children. We imagine they chose fathers to make sure that they knew these were men with "functioning" reproductive systems. They somehow persuaded all of these men to give a "sample." Then, they performed a semen analysis.

They found that the volume of their "emission" ranged enormously from about 0.1 milliliters to 11 milliliters. That's like a few drops all the way to more than a third of a small shot glass. The average amount of semen produced in one ejaculation was about 3 milliliters (mL), or just over half a teaspoon. But can anything change this?

Fast-forward to 2005. A study of more than 6,000 men providing almost 9,500 samples was conducted from 1995 through 2003. They found that the volume did increase gradually the longer a man went between orgasms. Men who had not ejaculated in seven days had an average semen volume of 3.7 mL. Men who had orgasmed the day before had a semen volume of 2.3 mL. That's a change, but this is really a small volume difference. It's less than a third of a teaspoon. It's not something anyone would be likely to notice. Even men who had come earlier that day still had an average volume of 2.4 mL, which was actually more than those who waited a day. In fact, the difference between coming twice in a day, and waiting three days was less than a quarter of a quarter of a teaspoon. We're talking drops.

But some people really want to make a splash. They'll try anything. Some believe that priming the pump will make a difference. Will it? Will your quickie produce any more or less than your lengthy sexual encounter? Let's go to another study out of Canada. Twenty-five men between the ages of twenty-two and forty-four were gathered together, and they provided more than 290 different specimens over a four-month period. They were told that they had to forego any ejaculations for at least three days before producing their contribution to the study. The scientists found that the time taken to produce an ejaculation was significantly related to the concentration of sperm in the ejaculate, but that it had no relation to the actual volume. This was confirmed in another study of 142 men in a clinic in Sweden in 2008. So slow down, speed up—it doesn't matter. It doesn't change how much you will come.

There's just not that much you can do. Moreover, even if you can make a statistically significant difference, it's not likely to be one you're going to notice in real life. Most men come less than a teaspoon. Shouldn't that be enough?

Start Small, Stay Small

No matter how many times people say that size doesn't matter, it continues to be a topic of discussion. Men are worried about it. Women are talking about it. We've already discussed some of the myths as to how people try to judge the size of a penis by looking at other parts of a man's body, be it their feet, their hands, or even their forearms. Faithful readers know that none of the prediction methods work. There's no way to judge the size of a man's penis by looking at some other part of their body.

What about if you catch a glimpse of a penis when it's still soft? Can you judge what size that penis will be when it gets hard?

A lot of people also worry that if a man's penis starts small, it will stay small. They assume that if a man's penis is small when it is soft, it will remain peewee-sized when it gets hard. And, the erect penis size is what people really care about when it comes to sex.

Could there actually be a study on this topic? Of course there is. In fact, there are more than you'd imagine.

The first big study was done by Masters and Johnson in 1966. They gathered together forty men whose flaccid (soft) penises measured between 3 and 3.5 inches and another forty men whose flaccid penises measured 4 to 4.5 inches. Then, they measured how much the penises lengthened when they became erect. What they found was that the smaller penises grew about 3 inches, while the larger penises grew about 2.75 inches. Not much of a difference, in fact not a statistically significant difference. But this meant that larger flaccid penises were likely to be larger erect penises.

This was a pretty small study, and it didn't have much of a range of size among the flaccid penises. So in 1988, researchers used Kinsey data to do a much more comprehensive analysis. They divided about 2,500 men into two groups: those with flaccid penis length 3.5 inches or less and those with flaccid penis length of 4 inches or more. The first group had an average flaccid length of 3.2 inches, while the second group had an average flaccid length of 4.4 inches. When the penises became erect, however, the differences narrowed. The first group had an average erect length of 5.8 inches while the second group had an average erect length of 6.5 inches. In other words, flaccid penises grew, on average, more than an extra half inch when becoming erect. To be thorough, they also examined the effect that height and weight might have on these measurements. Neither of these was associated with penis size at all, flaccid or erect.

To recap, this was a study of over 2,500 men. The average size of the flaccid penis was 3.9 inches, and the average size of the erect penis was 6.2 inches. The average circumference (if that's your thing) was 3.8 inches flaccid and 4.9 inches erect. And there is absolutely, positively no way that you can predict how far from those averages any man will be. Even if you see his penis when it's soft, you can't tell how big it will be when it's hard.

Don't Swallow Your Cum!

It seems like people spend an inordinate amount of time trying to come up with reasons not to swallow semen. In our previous books, we dismantled the myth that semen is high in calories. Since then, we've heard from plenty of you that there are many other reasons to avoid semen. One of them is that it's "dirty."

Semen is remarkably clean. In fact, the vast majority of the time, it's sterile. Of course, if a man has an infection, especially a sexually transmitted infection, then it's possible his semen might be infected. But if that's the case, then forget the semen—you don't want his penis anywhere near you, either.

As long as a man's genital area isn't infected, his semen is totally clean.

While we're at it, compared to saliva, almost anything seems clean. The human mouth is a relative cesspool, as we discussed all the way back in *Don't Swallow Your Gum!* There is a lot more reason to panic about another person biting you than there is to panic about semen. The human mouth is full of bacteria. Way, way more than you'd find in the average ejaculation.

We imagine that there are other ways to define "dirty." But on almost any metric you might choose, semen is going to win out over saliva. (This gives a different dimension to the "spit versus swallow" debate!)

We're not trying to convince you to put semen in your

mouth and swallow it. If you don't want to do that sort of thing, that's totally your right. If you want to do it, though, then you might as well know the facts. Semen won't make you fat. Semen isn't dirty. In fact, it's probably one of the least noxious fluids a body produces.

Semen does have one very, very important quality that should not be forgotten. It can absolutely, positively make you pregnant. While sperm are not "dirty," you cannot forget what they can do around an egg!

There's Always Semen When You're Screamin'

One of our friends told us a hilarious story about his early experiences with sex. As a seventh grader, he and a girl would sneak off at school once a week and make out in the back of the school auditorium. It came as a complete and scary surprise to our friend when, one day, this secret session led to a wet explosion in his pants. Although the sessions and the in-the-pants coming continued for weeks and weeks, he had no idea that men ejaculate when they have an orgasm. Someone should have filled him in that there's always semen when you're screamin'!

But, is that true? Can men have an orgasm without ejaculating?

We have to start by saying that the vast majority of men *cannot* have an orgasm without ejaculating. After all, men are evolutionarily designed to ejaculate. It's the circle of life, the "coming of age." There's no good biological reason for men to orgasm without ejaculation. Ejaculation is the primary reason for male animals to have sex, and most men just can't help themselves.

Some men, though, do have "dry orgasms." When a man has a "dry orgasm," it's usually because something is wrong. The body is not working the way it should. For instance, men who had a condition called posterior urethral valves in infancy are more likely to have a slow or dry orgasm later in life. This is because there is something inherently abnormal in their urogenital tracts. Older men who have undergone radical prostatectomy are also more likely not only to be impotent, but to sometimes have dry orgasms as well. The prostate makes most of the fluid that goes into ejaculate, and so taking out the prostate gland disrupts the system. Some men having dry orgasms report differences in sex, like they don't feel the "point of no return" when ejaculation seems inevitable.

Additionally, some drugs are associated with a higher rate of dry orgasm. Studies of certain drugs, like alpha-adrenergic blockers, used for benign prostatic hyperplasia, can lead to dry orgasms.

So the bottom line is that dry orgasms aren't impossible. This doesn't mean they are common. It also doesn't mean you should ignore them. As you would probably guess, men who suffer from orgasm without ejaculation often have a harder time fathering a child.

There are some reports of men who have trained themselves to prevent ejaculation with orgasm willingly and actively. Supposedly they have practiced stopping their urine midflow and strengthening the muscles that block fluid emission from the penis. Theoretically they can voluntarily stop ejaculation as they reach the "point of no return," allowing them to feel an orgasm without the accompanying release of semen.

But such reports do not appear in the medical literature (at least not where we can find them). So while we declare dry orgasm absolutely not impossible, it does seem unlikely—or at least really difficult—for men to stop ejaculating at will.

You're Going to
Break That Boner!

Just in case you haven't figured it out, a boner is not made of bone. A penis can get really hard, but that's due to its filling with blood. There are no bones involved. Does that mean you cannot break it? No.

Breaking your penis is so horrible to contemplate that it's even difficult to discuss. It sounds so terrible and painful that many just assume that it's impossible. And when it's flaccid, the penis is so obviously flexible and malleable that it seems almost inconceivable that it could snap. But penile fractures are real and, hard as it may be (sorry), we're going to tell you all about them.

We're not saying they are common, mind you. A paper reviewing six years of data in a hospital in Canada found thirty-four cases, eight of which also had damage to the urethra (the tube fluid exits from). About three-quarters of the reported cases happened during some form of intercourse. The penis must have snagged on something instead of going where it should have, it bent, and it broke. Another study, in Spain, found twenty-four cases over twenty years. Almost all of them occurred during sex. In the other cases, the cause was "penile manipulation." We'll leave that to your imagination.

Enough jokes. A penis breaking is rare (only about 1 in every 175,000 hospitalizations), but it's very serious. Most times, the men, and whoever might be with them, hear a popping sound, and feel something terrible when the penis bends and fractures. Immediate swelling, pain, and obvious deformities are usually present.

Most broken penises need surgery to fix them. Clots need to be removed, and sometimes the urethra needs to be repaired. After that, it's a period of "rest" when erections and activity is most certainly to be avoided. (Let your broken penis heal, people!) If they are cared for promptly, and instructions are followed, the vast majority of men go on to have normal lives after the incident.

Unfortunately, sometimes embarrassment or social norms prevent men from seeking prompt medical attention. That can significantly worsen the chances of a full recovery. If you think you've broken your penis—and we suspect you'll know—call 911 and get help immediately. You'll thank us later.

You Are Going to Pump That Geyser Dry

Has someone ever told you that you can run out of sperm? This myth is usually used by people who want to convince you to stop doing something. Maybe they think you masturbate too much. Maybe they think you are having sex too much. Or, maybe they think you're doing something wrong in trying to get pregnant. But the bottom line is that the use of this myth has one central belief: that you're wasting your sperm, because there's a limited amount of it.

It's not that we can't understand why people might think this is true. You are sending a lot of sperm out into the world every time you ejaculate. Every ejaculation contains hundreds of millions of sperm. A study looking at factors that affect the quality of men's semen found that a single ejaculation contains sperm in the range of 26 million sperm to more than 830 million sperm.

That sounds like a lot! Will your body be able to keep up with that kind of production? It's thought that the average man makes more than 500 billion sperm over the course of his life. Even so, blowing hundreds of millions of sperm per pop could make a man go through that allotment faster than he'd like.

But he can't.

Unlike women, who develop all of the eggs that they will ever make early in their lives, men don't start sperm production until they hit puberty. Then, their testicles start to churn them out at a pretty consistent rate. It takes a couple of months to develop the perfect sperm, though. They don't get made too quickly.

No one is sure of the exact rate at which sperm are produced. It likely is different for each man, and changes over time. But it's clear that millions, likely tens of millions are produced each day. Men are in constant sperm production.

When you ejaculate, a significant number of the recently developed sperm are released. If you ejaculate again shortly after the first time, it's clear that subsequent ejaculations will have fewer sperm, since fewer are available. But the number will likely never be zero. It takes a while, but you are more likely to run out of the other components of semen before you run out of sperm. You would likely have a dry orgasm before you have one without sperm.

Regardless, you keep making sperm continually. In a few days or even less, hundreds of millions will be available for your next ejaculation. Most men keep making sperm until they die, even if the quality of those sperm decreases with age.

If you're trying to get pregnant, then yes, you need to consider how to maximize your sperm. It's important not to waste multiple ejaculations each day before the one that counts. This is the reason why most doctors and health professionals will tell you to abstain, even up to a few days, to reach peak fertility. But you could masturbate like crazy for a full month, wait a few weeks, and your body would recover just fine. You would be back to full sperm concentration in your semen very quickly.

You can't "run out of sperm" in the long term. They are

constantly turning over. Unused sperm are reabsorbed, and new sperm are produced. In the short term, you can decrease the number available to fertilize an egg and get someone pregnant, but there's absolutely no reason to be worried about your long-term production or availability. Completely depleting your stores from overuse is a myth.

Part Two

WOMEN

Wearing a Bra Will Keep Your Boobs from Sagging

Both authors of this book hate wearing bras. We know you are shocked, but figured that we should disclose our biases up front. Nonetheless, we thought there were a lot of good reasons to wear them.

While many women wear bras because it is the socially acceptable practice within their culture or because they like how it looks, women have also heard that wearing a bra will keep their breasts in good shape or prevent them from sagging.

The idea seems to be that supporting the breasts will prevent the ligaments that support the breasts from becoming stretched out and allowing the breasts to sag. The breasts do not contain a lot of internal structure for support. They have a type of ligament called Cooper's ligaments, but the true function of those ligaments is not known. It is not clear that those ligaments actually offer the breast much support. Some experts think that the skin covering the breast might even be the most important part of supporting the breast.

Scientists and doctors do not actually know much about how to keep breasts looking good. While there is concern that letting the breasts bounce during high impact or repetitive sports stretches out what ligaments are in the breasts (hence the use of sports bras), the best type of brassiere to reduce the bouncing of breasts during athletic activities is still being investigated. (Bra scientists are urgently needed!)

Bras do alter how much breasts move, and they might have benefits for reducing discomfort from this movement. In a very small study of 3 women, wearing an external support (i.e., a bra) reduced the movement of the breasts during exercises that included running, jogging, marching, and walking. For these 3 women, wearing a bra also decreased the breast discomfort or pain the women reported, with the fitted sports bra doing the best at pain reduction. However, this is a very small study and is not enough to tell us about what happens for the entire female population. In another small study of 20 women with large breasts, the women had less breast discomfort and bra discomfort when they used a bra that both elevated and compressed their breasts, rather than a typical sports bra or nonsports bra. These bras did not actually change how much or how fast the breasts were moving when the women ran.

When it comes to everyday bra wearing (and not just bras for sports), there aren't any good studies to tell us whether bras actually make a difference. We really do not know whether wearing a bra helps, hurts, or makes no difference to the shape of the breasts.

One very small study of 11 women in Japan suggested that wearing a certain brassiere may have made the subjects' breasts tend to hang down more. Unpublished, "preliminary findings" from a sports medicine doctor in France also point toward this idea that bras may not be as helpful as people think. Dr. Jean-Denis Rouillon has reported "preliminary findings" related to fifteen years of following a reported 320 women and taking regular measurements of their breasts. (These findings are not yet published in a peer-reviewed journal, which means that we cannot evaluate how good the science really is. We can only let you know that this might be something interesting, but we want to see the actual data before we make any firm conclusions.) In Dr. Rouillon's study, the women went without bras for varying periods of time from several months to several years. Throughout the fifteen years and the time periods with and without bras, the women were asked about pain and discomfort. They also had their breasts carefully measured. Dr. Rouillon claims that the initial results "validate the hypothesis that the bra is not needed" and that "medically, physiologically, and anatomically" the breasts do not benefit from being supported with a bra.

Having proof that this is true would be a huge advance in our understanding of why women should or should not wear bras, but for right now we will need to hold off on drawing any conclusions. This is still a very small study compared to the number of women in the world, and the scientific methods cannot be examined until a paper is published.

So, we don't actually know whether bras will do anything to prevent your breasts from sagging. But we acknowledge that there are lots of other cultural reasons women wear them. It's up to you.

Women Don't Really Want Sex

For quite a number of years, much of the writing and science about men and women and sex has centered on the idea that men are hardwired to want sex and more sex, while women are more driven toward an emotional connection and babies. The theory is that women are programmed for monogamy for these reasons. Women might want sex because it leads to things, like love, but they don't just want sex for sex in the way that men do. You may have heard that women are not aroused by what they see, that women have weaker sex drives than men, or even that women's bodies are not designed for them to go after sex—only to receive sex.

More and more research has been accumulating to suggest that these ideas are all myths. While women's experience of desire, orgasm, and sex might differ from men's, much of how women's sexual desire is described and understood is shaped by what is acceptable culturally and socially. When it comes to the biology, there is plenty of research to suggest that women are also hardwired to have a strong sex drive in and of itself. In studies looking at women's responses to all sorts of sexual images and pornography (including men having sex with women, women alone, women having sex with women, apes having sex, and so on), women's bodies respond rapidly to all of these images. In fact, women often would not report that they responded to all of these images (particularly those that are considered less socially acceptable), but their bodies gave them away with strong reactions on all the monitors. Women want sex, too!

Although women may want sex just as much as men want sex, there are some differences in how relationships influence a woman's arousal compared to a man's. A study examining how women responded to audio stories describing sexual or nonsexual episodes involving either strangers, friends, or people in long-term relationships found that the women did not respond with as much sexual arousal to the stories involving either male or female friends. (In contrast, the men's sexual responses were not influenced by the relationships in the stories.) But this does not mean that women do not have as strong of sexual responses; they just respond differently to the context than men do.

Are women programmed to be monogamous? Actually, studies suggest that monogamy is rough on women, maybe even rougher on their sex drives than it is on men's sex drives. Studies point to the idea that women's libidos tend to go down when they are in a long-term relationship with just one person. In both studies in animals and in studies that survey women over long periods of time, having a lower interest in sex is correlated with how long they have been in a monogamous relationship. While some would say that this means the women have an easier time being monogamous because their sex drive has gone down, sex experts would say that this is not the healthy state for these women. The women are losing their desire to initiate sex or to have sex with their partners, which does not reflect sexual health. In a piece of good news for marriages and monogamy, the studies do also suggest that how well you get along with your partner and whether you have affection and a good fit between you will increase your chances of still desiring them.

Experts suggest that anatomy alone would indicate that women might even have more hardwiring toward promiscuity than men. The presence of the clitoris, an organ functioning only for sensation, and the ability to have multiple orgasms without a refractory period are both unique to women. The fact that women can have multiple orgasms without a recovery time in between may have been an advantage in evolution. If you can have one orgasm after another, this might promote having sex with multiple male partners in a short period of time. Having sex with multiple males would increase the female's chance of getting pregnant, which would then increase the chance of reproducing.

Over the years and in some cultures, the female sexual anatomy has been abused, modified, and even mutilated for these anatomic differences. We do not in any way condone these reactions to a woman's specific sexual anatomy and biology. Instead, we point out these amazing capacities in order to counteract the myths about women not being "wired" for sex.

Even if you are not quite ready to start thinking of yourself or the women you know as sexual creatures who actually have the anatomy and desire to go after sex with multiple partners in short periods of time, the most important truth here is that women should have a sex drive. Not having a sex drive is not a normal state of affairs. In fact, there are specific names given to these disorders, depending on what the problem is. The official names are hypoactive sexual desire disorder, female sexual arousal disorder, female orgasmic disorder, or persistent genital arousal disorder. If you are struggling with not feeling sexual interest or desire, not having sexual thoughts, and not having any responsive desire, that is considered a problem. This is not a normal state of affairs for women; this is a situation that should be addressed, likely with both your partner and with your doctor.

Bald Is Best (The Bush Versus the Brazilian)

Brazilian waxes. Clamscaping. Vajazzling. The world of pubic hair grooming is full of more options than ever for creating hairless and sparkling female genitalia.

In case you do not know what a "Brazilian" is (besides referring to someone from Brazil), a "Brazilian wax" is a procedure where wax is used to remove all of the pubic hair, including the hair over the labia and around the anus, or to remove all of the pubic hair except a small strip in the front over what is technically called the mons pubis.

Despite what you may hear, not everyone has gone the way of complete bareness (see the chapter on the myth, "Nobody Has Pubic Hair These Days"), but about 11 percent of women in a recent study in the United States do report that they are typically creating a hairless state around their genitalia. We could not find any studies describing how common it is to get "vajazzled"—a process whereby one has all of one's pubic hair removed, and then crystals, glitter, or other decorative items are temporarily applied to the genital area in a design of one's choice.

People might remove their pubic hair for a number of reasons. Some people think it is sexier for themselves or their partners not to have hair in the genital area. They may like to be able to see the genitals without anything else in the way or they may not like having hair get in the way during oral sex.

It may remind them of what they see in porn or create a somewhat different sensation during sex. Others say that being "bald" is not only more sexy, but also more clean and hygienic.

While sexiness is a personal judgment, anyone contemplating the removal of their pubic hair should know that there are actually some real risks involved. (You also might not be a big fan of the pain involved with having all of your hair in this very sensitive area ripped out by the roots, but we'll just assume that you are okay with that for now.)

One risk in removing the bush is the risk of injury during pubic hair grooming. Believe it or not, one study estimates that people in the United States had almost 11,700 injuries to the genital area between 2002 and 2010 because of pubic hair grooming. That's right! Thousands of people hurt themselves while trying to remove the hair from this delicate region.

Perhaps these injuries are not so surprising when you think about what people are actually doing in the quest for more bareness "down there." The most common ways to remove your pubic hair are shaving, waxing, electrolysis, or laser hair removal. In the largest survey of American women's pubic hair grooming habits, almost 70 percent of those who reported recent pubic hair removal said that they used shaving. And shaving is where things get dangerous! About 80 percent of the pubic hair grooming–related injuries are caused by nonelectric razors. The next most dangerous grooming tool is the scissors, followed by hair clippers. Razors, scissors, and hair clippers are sharp objects to wield in a very sensitive part of your body that you might not be able to see very well!

While it might sound slightly torturous, the hot wax used to tear pubic hair out from the roots is not quite as dangerous, causing only about 2.5 percent of the injuries.

Both men and women can get hurt with pubic hair removal; 36 percent of the injuries involved the external female genitalia and 34 percent involved the external male genitalia. The most common types of injuries were lacerations to these delicate parts (37 percent of the injuries), followed by rashes (33 percent), infections after trauma to the skin (16 percent), and abrasions (10 percent). Ouch!

Getting rid of your pubic hair can cause some other problems, too. The reason that we have pubic hair is essentially to provide delicate parts of our body with some added protection. For women in particular, the pubic hair protects the delicate folds and lips of the vulva from irritation or from being rubbed too much. Without pubic hair, the vulva is more prone to getting irritated, which can even result in a condition called lichen simplex, where the skin becomes thickened and irritated in a vicious cycle of itching and scratching. If you have not had pubic hair for a while, you can also develop lichenification of the vulva, where the skin or tissues get thick and leathery because of the long-term exposure to more friction.

Removing your pubic hair also puts you at a higher risk of some infections. A small study from France found that *molluscum contagiosum,* a common and very contagious virus that causes small wart-like bumps, was more common in women who waxed or shaved their pubic hair. Viruses, including molluscum and herpes, might be passed more easily from one person to another when more of the skin is exposed. Plus, both shaving and waxing can result in small areas of trauma to the skin. Even small breaks in the skin that you cannot see can allow viruses and other bugs to get into your system more easily. Ingrown hairs that can result from shaving or waxing can also get infected.

These infections related to pubic hair grooming can come from bacteria that are already in the area (especially those that live in and around the anus) or they can come from your sexual partners. If the salon doing your waxing does not use sanitary practices (say, for instance, that they reuse wax on customers or double-dip the wax stick into the wax after it already touched someone's skin), then that can increase your chance of infection. Without proper cleaning, bacteria, fungi, and wart- or sore-causing viruses can live inside of waxes, creams, and clothes, or on the salon equipment.

There have also been a few terrible cases of women getting very severe infections after Brazilian waxes. The state of New Jersey almost banned Brazilian bikini waxes in 2012 because two women ended up hospitalized with severe infections as a result of their Brazilian waxes. A medical case report from Australia also details how a twenty-year-old woman with type 1 diabetes developed a very severe bacterial skin infection with *Streptococcus pyogenes,* as well as the herpes simplex virus, because of her Brazilian wax. People with diabetes are more susceptible to infections, so this case highlights how pubic hair removal can be even more of a risk for anyone who has a weakened immune system.

On the other hand, Brazilian waxes might be ridding the world of one type of sexually transmitted infection—pubic lice! Pubic lice, which are sometimes called "crabs," require pubic hair or similarly coarse body hairs in order to survive. They actually attach their eggs or nits to the shafts of pubic hair or other coarser body hair like eyebrows or eyelashes. Historical data suggest that there are fewer cases of pubic lice in the world right now, and some researchers suggest that this coincides with the increasing trend since the year 2000 to remove pubic hair. We do not know the extent to which pubic hair removal might be responsible for this, in part because we do not have data for comparison about whether previous time periods or cultures where pubic hair removal was common had fewer cases of pubic lice. Physiologically, it does seem like a possibility, but the wonderful idea of being immune to pubic lice should be balanced against the risks of bacterial, viral, or fungal infections.

Obviously, almost anything that we do in life carries some risk with it. We are always making choices about whether we think the benefits of doing something will outweigh the risks. You might decide that the benefits of removing all of your pubic hair are well worth the risks of discomfort, injury, irritation, or infection. We want you to make an informed decision before you prepare to go bare.

G-men, G-spots—They Don't Exist!

It seems like we would be able to give you an answer on the G-spot without a problem. Yes, women have them—or no, women do not have them. Surprisingly enough, scientists, gynecologists, and sex researchers argue about this all the time. There are papers saying that all of the science points to women not having a G-spot and others that insist that women do have something along these lines. The opinions disagree so strongly that you could imagine these researchers getting into fistfights over the issue.

What is the G-spot anyway? "G-spot" is a term used to describe an especially sensitive zone that supposedly exists in a woman's vagina. This erogenous zone is supposed to be a sensitive area in the front of the vagina that can be stimulated to lead to pleasurable feelings, or even orgasms in some women. Among those who say that this spot exists, they suggest it is located on the front wall of the vagina, about halfway between the pubic bone and the cervix. The G-spot is often cited as being a source of "internal" or "vaginal" orgasms for a woman, as opposed to the clitoris, which can be stimulated for more of an "external" orgasm.

The person who earned the "G" in G-spot was Dr. Ernst Gräfenberg, a German obstetrician and gynecologist who did innovative work on female anatomy and sexuality back in the 1950s. In his words: "an erotic zone could always be demonstrated along the anterior wall of the vagina along the course of the urethra."

Two later researchers, Drs. John Perry and Beverly Whipple, dubbed this area the G-spot in Dr. Gräfenberg's honor in their 1982 book called *The G-spot: And Other Recent Discoveries About Human Sexuality.* They describe an area rather than a spot—an area on the front wall of the vagina that could be especially sensitive because a number of anatomical structures come together there: blood vessels, glands and ducts on either side of the urethra, nerve endings, the vagina wall, and the neck of the bladder. In their own study, 400 women were examined, and the G-spot was identified in each one.

You can also explore whether or not women have G-spots by—wait for it—asking women! Many, many women do believe that they have G-spots. In multiple large surveys, a majority of women report that they have G-spots.

Studies that look at the types of cells or human tissues support the existence of this area in terms of the various components coming together in one area. However, they also suggest that the composition of this area is somewhat different from one woman to another, which may be why it seems like some women do not have a G-spot or do not experience pleasure when this area is stimulated.

Contrary to popular belief, though, this potential G-spot area does not have more nerve endings than other parts of the vagina. In a study that took 110 biopsies from various areas in the vaginas of twenty-one women, there was no particular area in this region with lots and lots of nerves. While this small study could have just missed the spot, it is also supports the idea that the G-spot is not just a bunch of nerves, but a collection of other structures.

This all sounds fairly straightforward. Surely scientists can tell if a body part exists or not, right? And yet, there are still scientists arguing that there is no G-spot whatsoever, and that all of these women are wrong.

But the science supposedly disproving the G-spot is not particularly strong. One argument against the G-spot is that some scans, such as an MRI scan, have not revealed an obvious structure. The problem with these studies is that they usually only involve very small numbers of women. While scientists have argued based on one scan of one woman that they did not see a structure that they would call a G-spot, this does not mean that there is not a particularly sensitive area present. Another reason that some doctors argue against the existence of the G-spot is that women do not usually develop sexual problems after surgery is done on this part of the vagina. Studies actually show that women report better sex after these surgeries.

Does this mean that there could not have been a G-spot there? No. These findings do not mean there is no G-spot in that part of the vagina. The studies did not test the specific sensitivity of various areas of the vagina, nor is there any reason to disbelieve the women who are reporting better sex. Plus, the kinds of surgery that are done in this area repair sagging bladders or other problems causing incontinence. These women might report better sex because they are no longer incontinent!

The other argument against the G-spot has to do with the

idea that the entire area is quite sensitive or that the G-spot might be "in women's heads." Detractors say that, if you think that stimulating a particular area is going to feel good, then it will feel good. They think that women are imagining that they have a G-spot. Of course, this line of thinking could also be used to support the G-spot. Certainly, the brain is an important sexual organ. If you think something will be exciting or you think something will feel good or you want someone to touch you, that thinking should help you enjoy that thing! This does not mean that there is no sensitive area in the vagina; it just means that the psychology of sex might be the most important thing overall. Researchers both for and against the G-spot agree with that idea.

After reviewing the studies of the G-spot, it is clear that experts are divided and that the science is not rigorous enough to give us a clear answer. Much like with the science on female ejaculation (read the next chapter on whether women squirt!), the most rigorous studies do not show it happening or cannot explain where it is. However, public opinion (including the opinion of the women whose bodies are in question) is in favor of these things existing. Even though the strongest science may not support it, on balance of the data, we will come down in favor of the existence of the G-spot. (We're trying to be very scientific, but have to admit that there are likely some nonscientific reasons biasing this conclusion. We'll spare you the specifics. . . .)

Reasonable examinations have supported the existence of the G-spot, and no convincing science currently disproves these findings. One of the most important factors here is how important the brain is to the experience of sexuality. The reason to celebrate the G-spot is not because woman should be pressured to find if they have such an area and to have it stimulated. Instead, it should refocus us to know more about the parts of the body that can be involved in pleasurable experiences. If women are having orgasms and everyone is having fun, that's great!

Women Do Not Squirt Like Men

One of the amazing things learned by combing through the archives of sex research is that controversies can exist for hundreds—even thousands—of years on issues that it seems like we could easily put to rest. One of these is the question of whether women ejaculate, or squirt fluid, when they have an orgasm. Some women claim that this happens all the time, but people have been arguing about whether this actually happens for at least the last 2,000 years. Yes, that's right. Two thousand years!

Before we review twenty centuries of history involving women's orgasms, it might be helpful to have a quick anatomy lesson related to women's sexual equipment and men's sexual equipment. When men have an orgasm, they usually ejaculate or squirt out fluid at the same time as their orgasm. The sperm are produced in glands called the seminal vesicles. These glands also produce some fluid in which the sperm live (semen), and then the prostate gland adds fluid to this mixture as the semen is created and passes through on its way to the outside. This combination of sperm and fluid, known as semen, is spurted out at the direction of the man's prostate gland at the time that the man has an orgasm.

Women's bodies produce fluid to lubricate the vagina when they are sexually aroused, but they do not have an obvious equivalent to the prostate gland. While the penis and the clitoris are thought of as equivalents to each other in how they become erect and sensitive during sex, women's orgasms are typically thought to involve muscles contracting and relaxing and a pleasurable release, but not to involve the emission of fluid. In other words, many people don't think that women squirt when they come.

In contrast, many people across the years believed that women do squirt. Art and writing in both Eastern and Western traditions reference female ejaculation in various forms. Writings from China and India, including the ancient *Kama Sutra,* describe women emitting fluid or ejaculating during orgasm. Across the centuries, some of the same scientists who describe the "G-spot" also described female ejaculation. In the 1500s, a scientist named Reinjier De Graaf described female ejaculation and suggested that the glands around a woman's urethra (the periurethral glands) could be considered the female equivalent to the male prostate. For the last several hundred years, physicians have continued to debate whether women really can ejaculate. One of the most prominent more recent experts on the matter was Dr. Ernst Gräfenberg. Not only was the G-spot named after this Dr. G., but he published a report in 1950 on "The role of the urethra in female orgasm" that concluded that some women could, indeed, release large amounts of fluid from the glands around the urethra, and on his examination of these fluids, they "had no urinary character." If the fluid wasn't from these glands, another idea was that the bladder might fill with a liquid that wasn't urine, which was then released as pressure built at the time of orgasm. Some experts suggest this might still be the lubricating fluid coming from the vagina, just in a larger amount than usual.

Other scientists and physicians persist in the belief that any such fluid being released from a woman must be urine—in part because they doubt that the periurethral glands serve the same sort of role as the prostate and could release this amount of fluid. The most popular explanation is that women who squirt actually release urine from their urethras without realizing that's what the fluid is.

In a systematic review that attempted to put together all of the science on female ejaculation, they actually separated out two different ways that women might squirt. One was the "female ejaculation," where a smaller amount of whitish fluid would come from the periurethral glands, much like a female prostate. The other was closer to actual squirting, where a larger amount of dilute and "changed urine" would come from the urethra and bladder. They looked closely at "coital incontinence," which means leaking urine during penetration or during orgasm. In this review, they conclude that "fluid expulsions are not typically part of female orgasm," but don't reflect any problems with the system. In contrast, coital incontinence is something that should be treated because it could reflect a problem with the urethra being overactive.

There's only one real scientific study examining women's squirting through close observation, and it's a very small one. In that study, thirty-eight women were stimulated to have orgasms using vibrators, and scientists examined muscle contraction, nerve activation, and also the appearance of the genitalia very closely. During and after the time when these thirty-eight women had orgasms, no release of the fluid was seen from either the urethra or the vagina. The scientists concluded that female ejaculation does not exist, or that any fluid released is likely urine from women who might be prone to incontinence.

Is this the only evidence we have? What about porn? What about the Internet?

When you move away from the most scientific studies, reports suggest more possibilities. Pornography would lead one to believe that women can squirt fluid when they have an orgasm, but believe it or not, pornography is not science. When scientists try to re-create those experiences under scientific conditions, they don't see the same results.

Filling out surveys might give us a better idea of what happens in the privacy of the bedroom. When women are surveyed, as many as half report that they release some sort of fluid when they have an orgasm. Some think this fluid might be urine, but others report that the fluid is something closer to the fluid that men release during orgasm. A review of studies concluded that the large numbers of women reporting ejaculation is an overestimate—kind of like what happens when men measure their own penis length.

We could not find any studies testing what kind of fluid women release during orgasm. Remember, the only scientific study on the topic did not find any fluid being released.

A very small study tried to examine the question of whether women who ejaculate are having any other bladder problems. This study included six women who reported that they could ejaculate during orgasm and six comparison women who reported not being able to do this. They had the women track detailed information about their urinary symptoms and whether they had any other issues that would indicate a bladder or urethra problem or a tendency toward leaking urine in any situations. Based on this small, but detailed, comparison, the researchers did not find any reason to think that the women who could ejaculate were actually releasing urine or having any other issues with their bladders or with incontinence. They concluded that women who release fluid during orgasm can be reassured that they would not need further evaluation for bladder problems unless they had some other symptoms to indicate this was a problem.

Although the scientific studies are limited, the combined evidence suggests that some women can release or squirt fluid when they have an orgasm. Even though the most rigorous study on the topic didn't observe the phenomenon, large percentages of women report this happening when they have orgasms. Some sex researchers, such as Dr. Gräfenberg, have also observed this. The composition of this fluid is not well described. While not all women have this kind of fluid expulsion, there is the possibility that many do.

Blonds Have More Fun

Rachel secretly wanted this one to be confirmed by science. After all, the blond half of our myth-busting duo has plenty of fun, and she would have been happy to learn that her blondness gave her some sort of sexual advantage. It turns out that there may be some real advantages to being blond, but they have a lot more to do with sex thousands of years ago than with sex today.

Gentlemen may, in fact, prefer blonds. In a French study that experimented with waitresses wearing blond, red, brown, and dark-brown wigs, the waitresses wearing blond wigs received significantly larger tips from male customers. When it came to female customers, blonds didn't do any better with tips than any other hair color.

Is this true in places besides France? When you travel around the world like Rachel does, you quickly realize that blonds are much more common in some places (like the Netherlands, where Rachel's ancestors are all from) and less common in other places (like Kenya, where Rachel works and where her blond head sticks out for miles around). Other studies looking at human preferences have found that the preference for blonds is higher in places like France, where blonds are less common, than in places like England, where there are lot more blonds. Studies of magazines like *Playboy* also reveal that the women in those popular pages are much more likely to be blond than women in the real population.

The question of why blonds exist is an interesting one for scientists who specialize in genes and evolution. They have often wondered if blonds exist because of sex.

Natural blonds pretty much only come from one small part of the world; Northern and Eastern Europe have more diversity in hair and eye color. People whose ancestors come from there have a diverse set of genes that can give them lots of different eye colors (including blue, green, hazel, brown, and gray) and lots of different hair colors (from blond and red to brown and black). When you move out from that area and look at the rest of the world, the genes for hair and eye color are not nearly as diverse. You start to see only genes that give you brown eyes and black hair.

Did these freakish blonds and redheads appear in Europe because of chance variation in the hair color genes that evolved only in Europe? Or was something else going on— what scientists would call a force for selection—that would cause these genes to stick around and become more common? It turns out that if the hair color diversity was related to chance, it would have taken 850,000 years to develop the kinds of variety in hair color that are currently seen. (The mind boggles at how much faster the developers of hair dye can now assist in this process!) Since humans have only been in Europe for a mere 35,000 years, this means that some force besides chance must be pushing toward blonds and redheads. And what better force could be at work than sex?

The current conclusion among the geneticists and evolutionary biologists is that "sexual selection" is responsible for this unusual group of genes. "Sexual selection" means that creatures with certain genes are going to have more sex and thus reproduce themselves (and their genes) more often. Very visible hair is not going to help you with activities like hunting or hiding from predators (blonds are going to be picked off easily by the bears), so logic tells us that this strange, light hair must help you with breeding instead.

Across the animal kingdom, sexual selection does result in creatures with more colorful characteristics. Why exactly this happens isn't clear, but scientists think it may have to do with bright colors stimulating the brain toward sexual attraction, or even just the tendency to notice things that are brighter or stick out. The advantage to having hair that is a relatively rare color would help blonds and redheads to reproduce because, all other things being equal, you are going to choose to mate with someone who catches your eye.

From an evolutionary perspective, this could explain why blonds and redheads did pretty well in getting reproduced, despite how easily they might be spotted by predators or how they might have more difficulty hunting at night. The next question is why this would have happened in Europe and not in other parts of the world, and how this might occur more often for women than for men. The theories get pretty complex, involving the patterns of hunting and gathering dependent on weather, environment, animal population, and so on. The environment in Northern and Eastern Europe was one where men would need to hunt over large areas, and women would have fewer opportunities to gather food, thus needing more help from men. Under these conditions, men were more likely to get killed while they were off hunting, so there were less of them. And, the large distances the men were traveling meant that it would be pretty hard for them to take care of more than one wife in the way that men did in a lot of other parts of the world. This means that, in this particular part of the world, women were at a real disadvantage because there were more of them than men. This kind of tough competition is a good set-up for women who have unusual colors (like blond hair and blue eyes) to stick out more in the mating game, and for those unusual colors to become a real advantage. If there were plenty of men around, the competition wouldn't be so fierce.

Now, all of this is not to say that blonds really do have more fun. In fact, the current theory for why blonds even exist has more to do with a time 10,000 years ago when desperate women had fewer options, and may have had a better chance of getting someone to have sex with them if their appearance was more unusual. That's a pretty sad definition of fun.

There is no direct correlation between blond hair and having more sexual partners, more sex, or more orgasms. What is consistently correlated with having better sexual health, even in very difficult situations such as women who have had cancer of the vulva or have been victims of childhood sexual abuse, is being optimistic, having a positive outlook, and having more self-confidence. So, if blond hair makes you feel better about yourself or have a better outlook on life, you can consider becoming blond! Otherwise, this legacy of the happenings in a very small part of the globe thousands of years ago should play only the smallest role in your view of yourself or your potential sexual partners.

Nobody Has Pubic Hair
These Days

Pubic hair is a normal part of the entrance into adulthood. It shows that you have entered puberty, and adult genitals in their natural form are surrounded by pubic hair that grows in characteristic patterns—an upside-down triangle for women and a more diamond-shaped patch of hair for men.

While it is normal for the body to grow pubic hair, it is also normal for human beings to do all kinds of things to change or remove it. Pubic hair trends have varied over the years in much the same way that fashion, makeup, and other hair trends go in and out of style.

In art across various places and times, from ancient Egypt and Greece to the European Renaissance, nude women are sometimes depicted without pubic hair or with very little pubic hair. Theories for why women are painted and sculpted without pubic hair range from the idea that it may have been normal practice for some women in those cultures to remove their pubic hair, to the idea that male artists may have idealized the genitalia without pubic hair or even been afraid of what female genitalia might look like in their natural form. When we look at art, it's hard to know what average women and men were actually doing with their pubic hair, compared to what was being painted or sculpted.

What about women these days? Public discussions of pubic hair removal through waxing or laser hair treatments have become fairly commonplace, in part because popular media, such as television shows, can openly discuss these topics in many settings. Celebrity-focused Web sites feature bikini shots that suggest a woman needs to be hairless to stand up to scrutiny, and viewers of pornography say you have to look pretty hard to find any evidence of female pubic hair. Science even supports that claim! An analysis of photos of naked women featured in the centerfold of *Playboy* magazine between October 1953 and September 2007 reveals that the centerfolds from 2000 to 2007 were much more likely to have little or no pubic hair. Some college students report never having seen a woman with pubic hair. "Bald" seems to be the new norm.

Despite how common it may seem, not all women remove their pubic hair these days. How much you have depends a lot on how old you are, and to which groups you belong.

In a 2010 survey of 2,451 American women ranging in age from eighteen to sixty-eight, women were asked about shaving, waxing, electrolysis, and laser hair reduction. Among the 2,451 women, 11 percent of women removed all of their pubic hair most of the time, 20.1 percent of women did no hair removal at all, and the majority were somewhere in between. About a quarter of the women surveyed had removed their pubic hair at some time. While this means that pubic hair removal is fairly common, the results show that most women still do have pubic hair these days.

Women's pubic hair removal varied a lot with how old they were. Total removal of hair was most common among the youngest women: 20.6 percent of the eighteen- to twenty-four-year-olds and 12.4 percent of the twenty-five- to twenty-nine-year-olds reported that they were usually hair-free, while only 8.6 percent of the thirty- to thirty-nine-year-olds, 6.5 percent of the forty- to forty-nine-year-olds, and 2.1 percent of the fifty-plus year-olds reported typically being hair-free. This means that, at any given time, the majority of women in all of the age groups still had at least some hair on their genitals.

That study also paints a picture of who is more likely to be hairless. Women who removed all of their pubic hair were more likely to be younger, to have received oral sex (cunnilingus) in the past month, to be single with a regular sexual partner, to have looked closely at their own genitals in the last month, and to rate their genital self-image and sexual function higher.

A 2013 study from the United States looked specifically at pubic hair grooming habits among low-income women. In this study, they asked 1,677 low-income women about their practices related to shaving, waxing, trimming, or dyeing their pubic hair. They found that 66.2 to 86.1 percent of different ethnic groups practiced some sort of pubic hair grooming. These are higher numbers, but the study was looking at "grooming," not complete removal of hair. This study also found that white women were the most likely ones to be grooming their pubic hair, as were the women in the twenty-one- to thirty-year-old age group. Women who had had five or more sexual partners in their lifetime were also significantly more likely to be pubic hair groomers than those who had fewer partners. Women who were overweight or obese were less likely to groom their pubic hair, as were those who made less than $30,000 a year. How women groomed their pubic hair was also related to their ethnic group, with Hispanic women being more likely to use waxing than black or white women.

In a much smaller study involving 171 adolescents in Texas, 70 percent of the young women said that they usually shave or wax their pubic hair.

So, all of this research tells us that not everyone is removing their pubic hair. The removal of pubic hair is, indeed, growing in popularity, but the majority of U.S. women still have some pubic hair.

As to the men, we couldn't find any scientific data on how common manscaping has become. We'll keep you posted!

Little Lost Tampon, Where Did It Go?

Can you lose a tampon inside of you? In this chapter, we're just going to focus on the idea of misplacing something in the vagina. For questions about losing objects in other body cavities, go to the chapter on putting things in other places. (Don't put *that* in *there*!)

Lots of girls, especially those new to using tampons or new to the idea of putting anything inside of their vaginas, worry about losing that tampon inside. What if the string breaks? What if it gets too high up in the vagina? What if the tampon is stuck somewhere in your pelvis or belly for the rest of your life?

This myth of the lost tampon is easily debunked by anatomy. You cannot really lose a tampon inside of your vagina. The vagina is basically a closed tunnel. It does not open up into the rest of your belly. It can expand a lot, but it's a closed pouch. For anything to go anywhere else from there, it would have to go through the cervix. Unless a baby is coming out of it, the cervix only has a very, very small opening. Under normal conditions, the hole in the cervix is not wide enough to allow anything besides small drops of fluid, or tiny things like sperm, to get through. Tampons are not going to get through the cervix; neither is almost anything else you would stick inside of yourself. They're not going anywhere.

All of this being said, women *do* routinely forget about tampons in their vaginas. Or they may have tampons and other objects stuck inside of their vaginas much, much longer than they should be. Every emergency medicine doctor and gynecologist has had to remove a forgotten or "lost" tampon, or something else that got stuck higher in the vagina than the woman intended. Sometimes, more than one tampon is found inside the vagina, or these objects are not even noticed in there while the woman is having intercourse. The vagina can stretch out quite a bit (a baby can get through it after all!), and so forgotten things can stay inside of there. Adult women have been found to have bits of condoms stuck inside their vaginas. Younger girls tend to have things like toilet paper or small objects that they might have stuck inside—for exploration purposes—forgotten in there.

But forgetting something in your vagina, or accidentally getting something stuck in there is very different than the idea of losing something inside of you. These things are not lost; they are not going anywhere!

It's really bad to leave things in the vagina for too long. Foreign objects in the vagina cause irritation, get incredibly stinky and foul, and can cause serious infections. (The stinky and foul part should not be underestimated. Rachel is feeling a little sick to her stomach remembering her own adventures working in the ER and having to remove really terrible things from a woman's vagina.) One of the reasons that tampon boxes have a lot of warnings on them is that leaving a tampon inside for too long (where it absorbs blood and offers a great spot for bacteria to grow) puts a woman at higher risk of developing a very serious bacterial infection called toxic shock syndrome.

When something is stuck or forgotten inside of the vagina,

it may cause discharge, a bad smell, and some bleeding. You also may feel discomfort when you urinate or during sex, especially if the object is larger.

If you have a tampon or something else stuck inside of you, you may be able to get it out yourself. First, wash your hands with soap and water. Then, get into a good position for reaching into your vagina. Many women find it helpful to sit on the toilet and bear down like you would if you were having a bowel movement. Next, reach inside with one or two fingers, attempt to feel the object, and move it out. It is safe for you to reach inside of there. You may be able to reach the tampon string or to pull on part of the tampon itself. A partner also may be able to help you with this.

If you can't get it, or if it feels too uncomfortable, call your doctor. They have tools they can use to pull things out more easily. As we said, they do this kind of thing all the time. Even if you have something complicated inside of you, they will work to find the most comfortable and pain-free way to get it out.

You also need to call your doctor if whatever you had inside was in there longer than it should have been, if you are having any bleeding with it, or if at any time you are having discharge from your vagina. Your doctor will want to evaluate whether you need any antibiotics to treat an infection. They can also evaluate whether anything else is needed.

A Woman Needs Her Clitoris
Stimulated to Have an Orgasm

We will start right out by saying this is a complete myth. Women can have orgasms in all sorts of ways—through stimulation of their breasts or nipples, through stimulation or penetration of their vaginas or anuses, and also through the stimulation of their clitorises. Hooray for female orgasms! They come in many varieties.

There are even fascinating case reports of women with the amazing talent of reaching an orgasm when an eyebrow is stroked or when some other random part of the body is stimulated. Even more remarkable, there are a few women in the world who have spontaneous orgasms when absolutely nothing else is going on. This is not normal, but it is quite amazing.

You never know what part of the body might become sensitive enough to give you an orgasm. (Pay attention! Doesn't this sound like an excellent reason for fun experiments with a partner? All in the name of science. . . .) Orgasms from other areas of the body are often referred to as "zone orgasms." The upper thighs, the area of skin in front of the anus, the armpits—these are all zones from which some people have orgasms with the right kind of stimulation. There is also a case reported in the medical literature where a woman had orgasms triggered by her left foot! Again, you never know where it might be.

People who have had spinal cord injuries are usually paralyzed or numb from the level of that injury down the rest of their bodies. People with these injuries often find that the area of their body and skin that is right up above the level of their spinal cord damage becomes very sensitive. They will often be able to have orgasms from the right stimulation or stroking of the part of their body where sensation begins.

For many women, stimulating the clitoris really is the best way for them to have an orgasm. The clitoris is an amazing organ, the only part of the human body that is solely devoted to sexual pleasure. The clitoris fills with blood, swells, and stands erect when a woman is sexually aroused—very much like a small penis. (As the penis is also used for urination, the clitoris gets the special distinction of having a purely sexual function.) In a large survey evaluating women's sexual practices, 84 percent of women who reported that they had masturbated to orgasm had orgasmed through clitoral stimulation alone. For most women, the clitoris is the key to orgasm.

The other most common way for women to have an orgasm is through penetration or stimulation within their vaginas (i.e., having intercourse with a penis or having something else like a finger or toy inserted in their vagina). Again, 84 percent of females who masturbated to orgasm had depended on labia/clitoral stimulation, but 20 percent inserted something into their vagina.

Women often describe orgasms that result from vaginal stimulation as feeling different from orgasms that result from clitoral stimulation. This kind of orgasm is often referred to as an "internal orgasm" or a "vaginal orgasm." Some people think that an "internal orgasm" is of a higher quality or something that should be sought after instead of clitoral orgasms. The most accurate description is that they feel somewhat different from each other. If you only have one or the other, you might have fun experimenting with whether you can have the other kind, but you should not think you are lacking, incompetent, or having a lesser sexual experience if you do not have all manner of orgasms.

This is a good rule to follow with considering the other ways that women can have orgasms. Lots of types of orgasms are possible. Some women have orgasms when both the clitoris and vagina (and other sensitive parts) are stimulated at the same time. About half of women report distinct satisfaction from breast stimulation, and 11 percent stimulate breasts while masturbating. Some women have orgasms with anal stimulation. And some women have orgasms when other body parts are touched. This does not mean that all women will, or should, have orgasms in all of these ways, but it does reflect how varied and rich the sexual experience can be. Interestingly enough, brain scans actually show us that stimulating the nipples, clitoris, vagina, and cervix can all activate the same part of the brain. Furthermore, the odds that a woman will be satisfied with her sexual experience are the highest when you combine multiple types of sexual activity (meaning, if there was oral sex and vaginal intercourse rather than just one or the other).

Women's sexual anatomy is part of what makes the wide array of orgasms possible. Stimulating the visible portion of the clitoris may be the most obvious way to have an orgasm, but there are sensitive areas that include the labia, vagina, and cervix. In fact, in some cases, even women who have had their clitoris and labia removed can have orgasms.

On the other side of the spectrum, there are also quite a number of women who report never having had an orgasm. In The Kinsey Institute reports, a number of women report having only one or two orgasms in their lives, or worse, none. Given the many ways in which orgasms might be possible, these women just may not have found the right strategy for them and their bodies. Again, the fun of experimentation . . .

Another fascinating thing that studies of orgasms reveal is that what is going on in a woman's brain might be a lot more important than what is going on with her genitals. That sounds funny, but studies actually show that the direct stimulation of a woman's genitals is not as key to her ability to orgasm as is her ability to relax. Brain scans assessing the reaction to stimulation of the genitals of men and women by their partners showed that it's more important to men's orgasms that there be direct stimulation of the penis than it is for women to have direct stimulation of the clitoris. In fact, brain scans showed the differences between when women were really having orgasms and when they were faking them. During real orgasms, deactivation of the brain centers responsible for emotions like fear and anxiety occurred. This kind of deactivation of the emotional brain centers didn't occur when women were faking orgasms. Where men seemed to need touching of the genitals more than anything else, women in the study seemed to need this emotional deactivation even more. This may explain part of why a woman could have an orgasm without clitoral stimulation if the other circumstances are right for her arousal.

Buy Our Product for That Clean, Fresh Feeling!

There are some things that don't need fixing. One of these is, for lack of a better way to say this, the vagina. For a long, long time, females and their vaginas have been prospering, both in the animal kingdom and in the civilized world. But at some point, humans felt the need to introduce douching.

For the uninitiated, a douche is a device used to clean the vagina by rinsing it with water, or a water-based solution. It's based on the theory that the vagina is somehow dirty and needs cleaning. Of course, the vagina existed for a long, long time without the douche. We all seemed to get along just fine.

While many think that douching has been in the decline, a study from about a decade ago found that more than 22 percent of women douche, with over half of African American women reporting that they do. This is still a pretty common practice.

Does it work? Does it help? Well, there's almost no evidence that it does anything positive. Some women report that is makes them feel "cleaner." Some women, and we suppose some men, report that it can improve odor. Some people think that douching can prevent pregnancy by washing sperm out of the vagina after intercourse. There are no good studies proving that douching does this. Oh, and it's not going to prevent you from getting pregnant, so please don't use it as birth control.

In the anti-douche camp, there are a lot of good studies that prove that it's a bad idea. A recent study out of Egypt, where douching is common, found that it was associated with increased preterm labor and pelvic inflammatory disease. Another study from Turkey, which has a similar cultural attachment to douching, found that women were unaware of its potential dangerous consequences. A review of the evidence, published in 2010, showed that douching is associated with bad pregnancy outcomes including ectopic pregnancy, preterm labor and birth, chorioamnionitis, and low birth weight. These are bad things for mothers and babies! Furthermore, douching was associated with cervical cancer, endometritis, and an increased risk of sexually transmitted diseases.

Sometimes, we make light of certain practices because they seem silly and there's no good reason to do them. But this is one of those cases where it appears the harm significantly outweighs the potential, and unproven, benefits. Douching carries significant risk not only for women who do it, but also for the babies they may carry in pregnancy. Talk to your physician, and really think about not doing it.

Bigger Breasts Are Less Sensitive

When it comes to breasts, the current assumption tends to be that "bigger is better." This is a myth, of course, as many women would much prefer to have smaller breasts, and plenty of men are attracted to smaller breasts. In general, though, our current society seems to favor and promote larger over smaller. Certainly the booming breast implant industry would support this idea as well.

It might be because there is so much pressure toward bigger breasts being better that any justification for smaller breasts would be embraced and celebrated. One of the positive ideas about small breasts has to do with sensitivity. There is a widespread belief that smaller breasts are more sensitive than larger breasts. And having more sensitive breasts might translate into more pleasure for a smaller-breasted woman than a larger breasted woman.

There are even lots of theories why this is the case. Some have posited that larger breasts need longer nerves, and it therefore takes longer for the signals to travel to the brain. This nerve-length theory is a pretty easy one to debunk. First of all, sensations travel along the nerves remarkably quickly. Your reaction to having something crush your foot versus your hand is not going to be noticeably different. Plus, if this were the case, it would mean that men with smaller penises derive more pleasure from sex than well-endowed men. We rarely hear that argument! It would also mean that shorter men would be more sensitive than taller men. No one suggests these things. They're just not true.

It's important to understand that we're not talking about before and after breast reconstructive surgery. There is some good evidence to believe that after procedures, the skin can be less sensitive. That's true with many operations. Moreover, a loss of nipple sensitivity is a known potential complication with breast implants or reconstruction.

This idea specifically refers to natural breasts. People believe that naturally smaller breasts are more sensitive than naturally larger ones.

Interestingly enough, this might be a half-truth. The small-breasted women have some actual research on their side! In a 1998 study published by the University of Vienna, scientists gathered 150 healthy women and evaluated them—quite thoroughly—to see how their breasts differed in terms of sensitivity. The women were divided into three groups by breast size: small (smaller than 250cc), medium (250 to 500cc), and large (larger than 500cc). If you think in cup sizes, that's roughly equivalent to 32A or smaller, 32B up to 34C, and 36C and higher.

To test sensitivity, the researchers touched filaments to various areas of the women's breasts to see whether the women could feel them. The filaments were very fine, and they were testing for the ability of women to detect incredibly light touches. And, they found that women with smaller breasts could detect more light touches. If you go to the study, you can see that in the nipple, for instance, the "cutaneous sensitivity" was 2.9 in the small breast group, 3.1 in the medium breast group, and 3.5 in the large breast group. The smaller the number, the smaller the filament that could be detected (meaning the more sensitive the breast). This was a statistically significant difference.

But what the heck does 2.9 or 3.5 mean? We have no idea. But what we can say is that the definition of sensitivity in this study and the way most women care about sensitivity in terms of sexual activity aren't even in the same ballpark. This study was interested in if a woman could feel a hair tickling her breast with her eyes shut. When it comes to sex, that's not the main concern of most women.

There's no evidence that if a woman can more easily feel a tiny hair brushing her nipple that she will have more pleasurable sex that involves breast manipulation. None whatsoever. The actions of most men and women in bed involve far more pressure than this, and there's no data at all to support the notion that women with different breast sizes feel this kind of pressure differently.

We aren't telling you that it's wrong for women or men to prefer small breasts for a variety of reasons. And small breasts just might be a tiny bit more sensitive. But assuming you're going to enjoy sex more because of this sensitivity is a mistake.

That Hole Does Nothing for Me

Yes, we are talking about *that* hole. Many people believe that women can't have an orgasm through anal sex.

Have you read the chapter, "A Woman Needs to Have Her Clitoris Stimulated to Have an Orgasm"? If so, you shouldn't believe for a second that a woman would not have an orgasm through anal sex. Women can have orgasms in all sorts of ways! And while it might not be true for all women, women can have orgasms through anal sex. (Also of note, there may be much more fun ways for you to figure out that this is a myth rather than reading this chapter.)

During a woman's orgasm, both her vagina and her anus have regular contractions. This means that both the vagina and the anus clench and release over and over again. Among different women, the number of contractions and how long the contractions last can vary, but both the vagina and the anus are typically involved in the increase in pressure that occurs in the pelvis during an orgasm. In fact, scientists evaluating women's orgasms often use probes that measure pressure in both the vagina and the anus to do their measurements. All of this suggests that the anus is somewhat involved in any orgasm.

Penile-anal intercourse can absolutely lead to orgasms for women. In a study surveying about 10,000 men and 9,000 women in Australia, 0.9 percent of men and 0.7 percent of women had engaged in anal intercourse the last time they had sex.

While anal intercourse was not very common in this survey, "digital anal stimulation" (meaning, putting a finger in the anus) was much more common. More than 17 percent of men and 14 percent of women had experienced it the last time they had sex.

This study had two very interesting findings about what led to orgasms. It found that the more things that you did, the more likely you were to have orgasms—especially for women. If you had oral sex plus vaginal intercourse or touching plus vaginal intercourse, the combinations were more likely to lead to orgasms for women than vaginal intercourse alone. And if you did even more things than that, you had an even better chance that the woman had an orgasm. For men, at least 94 percent of them had orgasms with any combination that included vaginal intercourse. For women, the best bet for orgasms were with the combination that included the big three—vaginal intercourse, oral sex, and manual stimulation (86 percent reported orgasms) or with the dazzling duo of oral and manual stimulation (90 percent had had orgasms).

The other interesting finding for our myth-busting is that anal intercourse seemed to do well for orgasms. Although the numbers participating in anal intercourse were smaller, 91 percent of men and 70 percent of women who had had anal sex during their last sexual encounter reported that they had orgasms from it. That's right, 70 percent of the women had orgasms from anal sex. This does not mean that all women will enjoy anal sex, but it is a form of intercourse that some people do enjoy.

The climax to this story? Always believe that climaxes are possible. Don't disbelieve anal orgasms.

Part Three

SEX

Oysters, Chocolate, Bananas . . . Viagra?

Many people believe that certain foods are aphrodisiacs that will put you in the mood. Perhaps they dream that serving an unusual delicacy to that special someone will suddenly boost their chances of getting closer, or they envision their partner transforming into a beast of passion. For world travelers, Lonely Planet has even published a list of destinations where you can sample the world's best aphrodisiacs.

For millennia, human beings have believed that certain types of food or drink would lead to arousal. Oysters have been a favorite aphrodisiac since Greek mythology featured Aphrodite, the goddess of love, emerging on an oyster shell. Casanova was rumored to eat fifty oysters every morning to fuel his crazy sexual escapades. In the second century AD, Romans were writing about wine and oysters leading women into wild sexual behavior. Rachel adores fresh oysters (and wine, too). Does she need to be more cautious in her sampling of these shelled delicacies? (Aaron loves oysters, too, but the Romans did not seem to be too concerned about men's sexual debauchery. Go for it, Aaron.)

Chocolate is another favorite of Rachel's that is rumored to be an aphrodisiac. Women are typically thought to love chocolate, and some might assume that anything that makes a woman happy should be considered a top aphrodisiac. The allure of chocolate is not just a modern fantasy peddled by swanky chocolatiers with lovely confections wrapped in perfect gold boxes. Cocoa and cocoa products have been thought to have powers of arousal or healing for many, many years. The Mayans who first cultivated cocoa over 1,500 years ago not only thought cocoa was a drink from the gods (their art depicts a god with cacao pods growing from his body), but are also thought to have used it as a drink in religious ceremonies, as medicine, and as currency.

And then there are the herbs and plants. Traditional healers around the world have been using various types of plants to treat sexual disorders or enhance sexual experiences for thousands of years. From China and India to Rome and Greece, ancient healers have used plants including nutmeg, gingko, crocus, and lots of other types of plants to solve the world's sexual issues.

Among all of these foods, herbs, and special brews, is there scientific evidence that anything really works?

No study has ever showed any sexually enhancing effect from oysters. Nor can scientists find any special ingredient in the oyster that would suggest an ability to turn men or women into raging beasts. Oysters are mostly water, a few carbohydrates, and some minerals. They do contain a lot of zinc, which is a mineral that sperm need to be healthy, but otherwise there is no secret sexual ingredient in the oyster.

Many people speculate that the oyster has been seen as a sexual stimulant for so many years because its salty, liquid substance on a curved shell reminds those sampling them of the female anatomy. Over the years, other foods that might remind people of the male anatomy (bananas, asparagus, carrots) have also been rumored to be aphrodisiacs. You may not have been thinking of genitalia before you put that in your mouth, but now . . .

This brings up an important point: If a food makes a person think about sex—whether because it resembles the intimate anatomy or even because the person *believes* it might be an aphrodisiac—then that food might become an aphrodisiac. Our brains and the psychology of desire are the most powerful parts of our sexual experience. If you believe that a food will put you or your partner in the mood, then you will be in the mood. It works because you believe it will. If a food makes you think about sex, and that makes you want sex, then the food worked. That might make it an aphrodisiac.

You might still be wondering about other foods and herbs on this list, and whether their effect is in only your mind or whether they contain anything else that might make a difference.

There is no doubt that chocolate is a magnificent substance. Chocolate contains a lot of flavonoids, and flavonoids in general have antioxidant properties, which are good for the body. Several studies suggest that chocolate is tied to lower blood pressure and better functioning of blood vessels. Cocoa also increases nitric oxide in the bloodstream, which creates the kind of dilation of blood vessels that is needed for a man to have an erection. Lower blood pressure and better working of the blood vessels might have a positive effect on the male sexual equipment, keeping the penis working well for erections.

Chocolate has another effect that might contribute to why people like it so much, and which also might be stretched into an aphrodisiac effect. Chocolate can stimulate a small release of phenylethylamine and serotonin into our systems. These are natural chemicals that boost our moods or are released when we are in happy or pleasurable situations. Chocolate even seems to activate some of the same receptors in the brain as marijuana. This might be a way that chocolate works as an aphrodisiac: People who are in better moods may want to have more sex!

In addition to all of these ways in which chocolate acts directly on your brain, it also can have a psychological effect as chocolate is associated with comfort and romance in many cultures. If chocolate has these positive connotations for you, then it may also serve as a psychological aphrodisiac. So many reasons to love chocolate. . . .

There is also quite a collection of studies looking at all of those plants and herbs that have been used to help with sex over the years. One review pulled together all of them—whether done in a laboratory, tested in animals, or even tested in humans—to see whether there is evidence that any of the plants work. Most of the studies looked at the effect of various plant compounds on the sexual behaviors of rats, including how often the rats mounted other rats and how often they ejaculated. Quite a number of the plant compounds did increase how often rats or mice had sex or ejaculated, suggesting that these unusual medicinal plants could improve sexual activity. For rats, anyway. For example, *Curculigo orchioides* increased rat penile erections and rat penis weight. *Litsea chinensis* increased "penile erection index, mounting, and ano-genital sniffing" in rats. That's right—if you want more rat bum-sniffing, give them *Litsea chinensis*! Only one of the forty-one plants tested was tested on humans (where it had no significant effect). While some of these plants are edible in some form (roots, bark, leaves, etc.), none of these plants are things people normally eat. Until they come up with forms of these plants or herbs that are safe for testing in humans, we would recommend leaving the roots, bark, and leaves to the horny rats.

Even though certain foods have been thought to promote sexual activity for hundreds or thousands of years, there is no scientific evidence linking any one food to enhanced sexual desire or pleasure. On the other hand, if you like those foods, there's no reason not to eat them!

Don't Put *That* in *There*!

Have you always secretly imagined what it would be like to put *fill-in-the-blank body part* into *fill-in-the-blank opening*? (Fill in the blanks with your body parts and cavities of interest!)

When it comes to body parts and sex, human beings have tried out pretty much every combination that you can imagine. Penises in vaginas, mouths, and anuses are among the most common sexual practices to "fill in those blanks." Fingers or hands inside of vaginas, mouths, and anuses are also very common. Some people also like to put things into urethras—that means into the male penis or into the urinary tract opening of a woman. You are, by no means, the first person to have done or thought about doing any of those things. In fact, we have thousands of years' worth of art in the forms of pictures, writings, and sculptures showing us that humans were doing and thinking about all of these things for a long, long time.

The advantages to human beings having had sex for so many thousands of years (besides the continued survival of our species) is that the historical example should be very reassuring to you. Other people do these things all the time and people survive, no one gets hurt, and hopefully everyone involved has fun. Penises and fingers fit into vaginas, mouths, and anuses just fine, and if you are interested in trying out those combinations, there are lots of ways to do that safely and enjoyably. Hands can also fit in vaginas, mouths, and anuses, although there may be a little more work involved in making sure that the practice is safe and enjoyable.

Do you really think you are the only one? Come on. For example, in conservative estimates, 30 to 40 percent of American women have had anal sex. On the other hand, 80 percent of Americans surveyed could not tell you the right answer to how many women have had anal sex.

Now, things do occasionally go wrong. Very rarely, these practices can even go horribly wrong. But these problems can usually be averted through pretty basic precautions, including the all-important need to do these things only with other consenting adults.

What do you need to know before you put *that* in *there*?

First of all, you need to know some basics about infection risks. Sexually transmitted infections, including HIV, herpes, gonorrhea, and human papillomavirus, can all be transmitted between penises and mouths, penises and vaginas, and penises and anuses. They can even be transmitted between hands and mouths, penises, vaginas, or anuses if bodily fluids such as blood, semen, or vaginal fluids are involved. The best way to prevent these fluids from infecting your partner is to use something like a condom (male or female versions) or a dental dam to create a barrier that any infected fluids could not cross. Even condoms are not perfect at preventing all infections from spreading, but you are much, much safer if you use a condom than if you do not use anything at all.

All of the sexually transmitted infections are also more likely to infect you if there is any bleeding or tearing of the tissues in the area. This kind of damage, even when it is not serious or does not cause pain, breaks down the barriers that the body naturally has to prevent viruses or bacteria from causing a new infection. Because you are more likely to have small tears or bleeding when you put things into new places or stretch something in a different way, you can sometimes have a higher risk of contracting a sexually transmitted infection.

Making sure whatever body part is being inserted is clean, washed off, dried, and free of any sores or fluids is also a good precaution. A clean body part is second best to condoms or barriers for preventing sexually transmitted infections. Other germs can be passed on from one part of your body to another if you do not clean off the body part being inserted. In particular, you should remember that the anus and rectum are the home to fecal bacteria that should not normally be inside of the vagina, urethra, or mouth. If you have put something into the anus, inserting that same body part into the vagina or mouth or near the urethra without cleaning the body part off runs the risk of giving your partner a bacterial infection.

You also need to consider whether something fits comfortably, and this may vary from person to person. While it is often fairly easy to determine whether something is too big, years and years of human experience also reveal that certain openings are remarkably adaptable. In particular, the vagina and the anus and rectum are very good at stretching.

In fact, the vagina has an amazing capacity to stretch, as demonstrated by its ability to have a human baby pass through it successfully. However, you need to remember that the female body changes in special ways during pregnancy to make it possible for something large to fit through. During pregnancy, the body releases hormones that actually soften the tissues of the birth passage over time to make it possible for something as large as a baby to get out. When a woman is not pregnant—or even when she is early in pregnancy—the body has not made these changes, and you might not be able to fit something as large. If you try to put something too big into the vagina, it could result in pain and bleeding. On the other hand, the vagina usually has no trouble accommodating something like a large penis or an entire human hand or fist, especially if this insertion is done carefully and gradually.

The anus and rectum are also very good at expanding; however, the anus does have a sphincter—a tighter, muscular ring meant for contracting. There is a limit to how much that sphincter ring can stretch. When you get beyond the limits of the sphincter, there will be tearing—even though the rectum past that sphincter can stretch quite a bit more.

The most important consideration in your exploration is that all of the involved sexual partners should be comfortable with what is going on, and they must be consenting adults. The basic advice is to start with something of smaller size and to gradually work your way up to something bigger. It's also a good idea to insert things slowly and gently, especially the first time that you are trying to insert a particular body part in a particular body cavity. Lubricants that are safe for use inside of the body are also very helpful for getting something inside without pain, bleeding, or tearing.

The same suggestions apply if you are trying to put more than one thing in more than one opening at the same time. Attempting to involve more than one partner at the same time, or to use both two parts and other objects at the same time, can be done, but it's done most safely with smaller items, slow entry, and lubrication. The added pressure of having something in both the vagina and the rectum at the same time can lead to a higher chance of tearing the tissues, so you do need to be careful.

While the amazing stretching ability of the vagina and rectum answer a lot of the questions about whether it is okay to put a particular body part into them, there are still some examples that should caution us that things do occasionally go wrong with some of these activities. There are many terrible cases in which rape or sexual assault is so forceful that it tears a hole through the walls of the vagina or rectum. Obviously, this causes tremendous pain, and can also result in bleeding, infection, and even death. When a partner is unwilling, their body might sustain more trauma because the vagina or anus is not able to relax, or because there might be less lubrication than normal. The risks of having an injury as a result of putting a body part into a body cavity are also much higher when children are involved, reinforcing the rule that those involved with these practices must be consenting adults.

There was also at least one tragic case in which a sexual partner inserted his hand into the vagina of a young pregnant woman in a way that forced an air bubble up through her cervix and into her bloodstream. This bubble (what doctors would call an air embolus) killed her. Although this was a very unusual case, this is a reason why doctors caution pregnant women about sexual activities that involve air being blown or forced into their vaginas.

You might also have questions about whether it's okay to put something that is not a part of your body into one of the cavities or holes of someone's body. Once again, part of the answer lies in the fact that human beings have tried more things than you can probably come up with in your wildest imagination. Humans have inserted everything from sex toys to household items to food to small animals to drugs into vaginas, anuses, and urethras. ER doctors can tell you all kinds of stories about the crazy things that they have found or heard of having been found inside of people's bodies. While some of these stories are likely apocryphal (there are no published medical reports of gerbils in rectums, for example, but the stories of celebrities indulging in this practice are fairly common), human beings have experimented with all sorts of insertions. If you want to see lots of X-rays showing the crazy objects doctors have seen in peoples' bodies, refer to the great book, *Stuck Up! 100 Objects Inserted and Ingested in Places They Shouldn't Be.*

Most of the time, these experiments work out just fine. Again, there are a few simple rules to remember. First, size and comfort are key issues to consider. You also should not insert something with a sharp edge or point into any of the body's orifices as cuts, lacerations, and punctures can all result in bleeding, infection, and even death. Second, you need to be able to remove the thing that you are inserting. It might be a lot easier to push something in than to get it out, so the best course of action is to make sure you are holding on to it the entire time. Things don't get lost inside of the body (the reproductive tracts and the gastrointestinal tract are essentially closed off), but you might have to make an embarrassing and physically uncomfortable trip to the ER if you need help to get out whatever you have put inside. Third, you should think about the infection risk. Foods, plants, and anything that rots can serve as food for bacteria and lead to infections. When you eat these things through your mouth, your body usually breaks them down very, very well before they get to the end of your digestive tract. That means that it is not necessarily safe to put something inside from the bottom even if it would be okay to swallow it from the top.

Also, the same bodily fluids that carry sexually transmitted infections when they come from your genitals (semen or vaginal secretions) and blood can cause infection when they are introduced on other items. For example, there is a case report of a woman who was infected with HIV by blood-tinged vaginal secretions on a sex toy. When bodily fluids of any sort are involved, you have to think about infection risks. Any toy or other item should be washed with soap and water and dried off completely before it is put inside of the body. An antibiotic hand sanitizer is not enough to clean off all bacteria, particularly a stubborn kind of bacteria called *Clostridium difficile* that can come from the rectum and cause infections.

Not only should you avoid putting inside things that can rot or get stuck, but you also need to consider the potential for irritation or allergies. The vagina and rectum are both accustomed to their own set of fluids and germs. When you put new things inside those places, it can causes rashes, irritation, changes in the normal bacteria that keep the area healthy, and other infections. Scented lotions or soaps can especially irritate the urethra, vagina, and rectum, which makes it a good idea to only use lubricants that are safe for use inside the body. Plain petroleum jelly or a lubricant designed for this kind of personal use are less likely to cause problems than foods or other lotions.

When you think about things you would like to put inside the body, you also may be thinking that bigger means better. But the vagina only has the kind of nerve endings that give you most sensation (somatic sensory innervation) in the lower half or third. Things that extend up further inside the vagina may not create much more sensation. Most of what you feel when something is inserted through the anus comes from the area that is right around the opening, from the area of that sphincter. When objects go much higher in the rectum and into the colon, different kinds of nerves are involved and they are usually much less sensitive to being stretched or filled up.

In summary, it is okay to experiment sexually with a lot of different combinations of body parts and objects. You can probably put *that* in *there,* and it's almost certain you won't be the first to do it. But your experiments will be much safer— and likely more enjoyable—if you follow the principles of only involving consenting adults who are comfortable with the process, starting smaller and slower and working your way up in size, using protection or keeping things clean, and assisting the mechanics with lubrication.

It Will Really Turn a Woman On
If You Do the Laundry

You may have heard that the way into a woman's heart is really through a little housework. Picking up those dirty socks, doing the laundry, washing the dishes, vacuuming . . . surely nothing will turn her on more than helping out around the house.

After all, women still do a *lot* of housework. Studies show that women do much more than men, or about 70 percent of the work around the house. Men's contribution to housework is on the rise though. Men have gone from doing 15 percent of the work in 1960 to 30 percent of the housework in 2003. It is not a big stretch to imagine how a 50/50 split would leave women with more energy and time to get excited about their partners.

More equity around the house might indeed be a good thing for a marriage. Studies have connected men doing more housework with women feeling that things are fairer in their relationship, and with women having greater satisfactions with their marriages. And marital satisfaction is correlated with sexual desire in some studies, so perhaps housework will lead to satisfaction and satisfaction will lead to more desire.

One survey does support the idea that doing the laundry will score you some serious points in the bedroom. In a book in which the author interviewed 300 couples, the author identified that sharing housework more equally among men and women was linked to happier partners, with less need for marriage counseling and fewer divorces.

This is a great idea—and truth be told, we are all for equality in sharing the work—but the interviews with 300 couples do not represent the best science on the subject. It describes a relatively small group of people, and they were not studied in the systematic method of a scientific experiment. Recent studies that look at much larger segments of the population suggest that this great idea might not be true, at least when it comes to the amount of sex. Men who do more work around the house might actually have less sex, not more sex.

First of all, time does not seem to be the real issue. How often couples are having sex does not decrease when they are both working full-time or when they are spending more hours working. In fact, spending more hours in housework and paid work is actually connected to having more sex in one study. (Work hard, play hard!)

Even if time is not an issue, housework itself might still be an issue. Or it might signal other issues that are related to how often you have sex. Looking at the National Survey of Families and Households, which uses data that are almost twenty years old, but represents a much bigger sample of the American population, households with a more traditional divide of housework in which women are doing more of the work were also the same households that had more sex. In this study of over 3,500 couples, the difference in how often the couples were having sex could not all be explained by how happy the couples were (or were not); the housework divide alone seemed to make a difference.

For couples where the man did a larger than normal amount of the housework, the couples also had a lower frequency of sex. The frequency in sex continued to go down with the more "core housework" the man did. Core housework was things like cooking, washing dishes, cleaning the house, and doing the laundry. In contrast, if the man did more of the "man-typed tasks" (things like outdoor work, paying bills, car repairs), then the couple also had more sex. Husbands who did all of the man-typed tasks actually reported 18 percent more sex than couples in which the man did none of the man-typed tasks. It seemed to be the gender-typing of the role, rather than the work itself, that was most closely tied to having more sex; the men who played more of a "typical man role" were also having more sex. Just how these gender roles play into the divide of labor and the frequency of sex is not completely understood, but it is that kind of difference that the study points to.

Does all of this mean that you have an excuse not to do the laundry? No. Your partner might still be a lot happier if you have an equal split of household tasks, but it is possible that there are other things going on in such a relationship, things that might be connected with having less sex, like a reluctance to have sex with a wife who does not want to have sex with you. Plus, it bears remembering that these data are twenty years old and things may have changed significantly since then.

Remember our chapter about what women do want? The good news in all of this is that women do want sex—whether or not they are with men who are doing the laundry or not. And in a long-term relationship, a woman is more likely to continue wanting sex if she is satisfied with the relationship. There's plenty of room for exploration here.

Don't Leave Your Socks On!

This myth seems like a no-brainer truth: What kind of lame sex are you having if you, or your partner, don't even bother to take off your socks? Surely the whole point of the phrase "knock your socks off" would imply that a good time in the bedroom means the socks are coming off.

Interestingly enough, a study examining orgasms in men and women suggests that there may be very good reasons to leave your socks on. A sex study in the Netherlands did brain scans on men and women while their partners attempted to give them orgasms by stimulating their genitals. Apparently, it was quite drafty in that scanning room, and a lot of the study participants were complaining about having cold feet. (Actual cold feet—not just regretting their decision to participate in a study where they had to try to have an orgasm while their head was strapped down for a brain scan!)

When the study participants were given socks to keep their feet warm, significantly more were able to have orgasms. While the scientists conducting this study were primarily focused on describing exactly what happens in your brain when you have an orgasm, they also reported that in their unpublished findings socks were associated with having orgasms! Eighty percent of the participants who were offered socks were able to have orgasms, whereas only 50 percent of those who were not offered socks could have orgasms. Warm feet made it more likely that you would be able to come. You may not think that socks are the sexiest look for sex, but if socks make you so much more likely to be able to have an orgasm, you might want to try them the next time your cold feet are distracting you.

While the feet are certainly an important and sensitive part of the body, this study points at an important, larger issue about sex. The best sex may happen when you are comfortable. What this comfort looks like can vary from person to person. Comfort may mean warm feet, it may mean sex in a place you find relaxing, and it may mean a partner with whom you feel the most secure.

It may be especially important for women to be comfortable. The same study from the Netherlands found that "deactivating the emotional brain centers" (in other words, relaxing and releasing anxiety and worry) was at least as important for women during sex as having their genitals directly stimulated. While genital stimulation was most important for men, women essentially needed their conscious brains to be able to shut off to have a real orgasm. And socks might help you do that!

Lose Weight Fast! Have Sex!

Who doesn't love the idea of sex as a workout strategy? Imagine—have fun, have orgasms, burn calories, and get in shape—all at the same time. Perfect!

Sex does burn calories. Experts estimate thirty minutes of sex burns 85 to 150 calories. Those calories could add up if you are having sex often enough. Theoretically, you need to burn about 3,500 calories to lose a pound of body weight, so if you were using up 100 calories every time you had sex, you could lose one pound if you had sex thirty-five times. That sounds pretty good. If you had sex more often or for a longer period of time, you could burn even more calories.

The problem is this: Most people are not having sex for thirty minutes. Instead, the average duration of sex is closer to five minutes. (See the chapter, "You Don't Last Long Enough.") In fact, the biggest increase in your heart rate and blood pressure during sex only occurs for about fifteen seconds during orgasm, and then things quickly return back to normal.

Plus, you probably do not work as hard as you think you do while you are having sex. Based on studies of young married men, the amount of stress on the heart during sex or the increase in the heart rate is estimated to be about the same as walking up two flights of stairs. It is considered mild to moderate physical activity, and your heart rate rarely increases above 130. Yes, you are doing something, but it's not enough to count as a real workout. Of course, it's possible that if you have to work a lot harder to have an orgasm, or if you are older, or not physically fit, sex might entail a bit more strain for you.

Unless you are having sex for much longer and with much more vigor than is average, sex alone is probably not going to get you anywhere near the recommended amount of exercise. The current recommendations for an adult to be healthy are to aim for two-and-a-half hours per week of moderately strenuous physical activity. This would be the same level of effort as brisk walking or dancing. If you think you can achieve this with sex, by all means go for it, but most people are just not getting enough to reap all of the benefits of exercise.

To Be or Not to Be . . . Pierced

The popularity of piercings in the most sensitive of places has risen and fallen across the centuries. There are references to penis piercing in documents as old as the *Kama Sutra* (which dates to sometime between the first and sixth centuries AD). A particular type of penis piercing is referred to as a "Prince Albert," in reference to the husband of Queen Victoria of England. The prince was rumored to have a penis piercing that was intended to help straighten out his penis. In the last twenty years, body piercings of all varieties have become more popular once again.

Piercing the genitals of either women or men is often thought to be more common among sadomasochists, homosexuals, or people with fetishes, but there is not much science to back this up. The 1983 study that most supported this idea merely looked at what kinds of advertisements were placed in magazines for people who were very into piercings, and they found high rates of advertisements related to sadomasochism or homosexuality. The study did not look at the actual behaviors or desires of the people with the piercings.

In more recent studies, less than 20 percent of people with piercings reported that they saw themselves fitting the description of a masochist, sadist, or fetishist. Body piercing is more often described as a "body project" or a statement of one's personal identity. Even if body piercers do not fit these more extreme categories, there may be certain personality traits that go along with piercings. Body piercings, with or without tattooing, have been associated with other risk-taking behaviors.

One of the largest studies to look scientifically at the issue of who gets pierced interviewed a group of almost 1,000 people in New Zealand who had been followed since the time of their birth. When this group reached their twenty-sixth birthday, they were asked about both body piercings and their sexual behaviors, and this information was compared to assessments of their personality traits that had been done a few years before. Of the 966 people they could interview, 9 percent of the men and 29 percent of the women had piercings at sites other than their earlobes. Only 0.8 percent of the men and 0.6 percent of the women had genital piercings, so those were still fairly uncommon. In the analysis of personality traits, piercing was more common among women who had "low constraints" or "high negative" emotionality, but there were not personality characteristics tied to men with piercings. Women with piercings were also more likely to report having five or more heterosexual sex partners, same-sex attraction, and having any same-sex partner in the last year. The men's reports of sexual behaviors were not different between the pierced and nonpierced groups. The scientists who conducted the study thought that the combination of the women's piercings, behaviors, and personality traits might reflect that piercing was another way in which this group of women expressed themselves through their bodies.

Several small studies have assessed women with genital piercings, and how they view these piercings. In interviews with two women with clitoral rings, both women described how the piercing acted as both body art and also as a way to enhance their sexual arousal. Another study compared women's responses before and after piercings of the clitoral hood: 77 women were asked to complete questionnaires, but only 33 filled out all of the information before and after their piercings were done. Among this group, the level and frequency of sexual desire reported were higher after the piercings compared to before the piercings, but they didn't have any significant changes in how often they had orgasms or how satisfied they were with them.

In a study of 240 women ages seventeen to sixty-one years with genital piercings, the women reported that they had got these piercings for both personal and sexual expression, and that these piercings were usually done after careful consideration—lasting two years on average. These women described the piercings as a normal and meaningful part of their lives, and 97 percent reported that they would get a genital piercing again. In this study, relatively large numbers of the women reported having experienced abuse (over half) and almost half had been told that they were depressed at some point. In interviews, many of the women reported experiencing empowerment and increased confidence because of their genital piercings.

People pierce themselves for all sorts of reasons, but most of them seem to do it as a way to enhance their general sexual and bodily experience. Less often do they describe connections to more extreme sexual behaviors. Rather than a cringe-inducing impulse, piercings are often a decision made with a great deal of care and consideration.

Methuselah Had Sex
Ten Times a Day

Everyone likes good reasons to have more sex. And what could be a better reason than the idea that sex will make you live longer? This is almost as exciting of an idea as thinking that having sex will help you lose weight or get in better shape.

We are happy to report that there is at least some truth to this idea. (And there was much rejoicing!)

You cannot draw a direct line from having sex to living longer, in part because we cannot set up the kind of study that would test this by forcing people randomly into groups where they could either have sex or not have sex and then seeing how long they lived. However, we can see that being sexually active is associated with or connected to a number of good things for health.

In large studies that examined over 6,000 adults in the United States, being sexually active, reporting higher quality of sex, and being interested in sex are all associated with good health. Those in good or excellent health reported more sex (having sex once a week or more) and being more interested in sex. The challenge with these studies is that they are not designed to say which thing causes the other thing. Does being healthy mean that you can go out and have more sex? Perhaps, but it is also possible that having more sex is keeping you healthier. The studies can't tell us which is going on. Either way, it is nice to hear that good health and sex are closely linked for adults across the lifespan from twenty-five to eighty-five.

The classic study quoted to support the idea that sex helps you live longer comes from 1982. Researchers followed 252 patients over the course of twenty-five years to look at what factors predicted who would live the longest. This study actually tells us that not only does sex matter for living longer, but it matters how good it is—and it matters whether you are a man or a woman.

Three factors were significantly tied to longer life: 1) frequency of sexual intercourse, 2) past enjoyment of intercourse, and 3) present enjoyment of intercourse. Interestingly enough, these factors were not the same for men and women. The frequency of sex was a significant predictor of living longer for men, but not for women. The enjoyment of intercourse, both past and present, was a significant predictor of living longer for women, but not for men. Having more sex is connected to men living longer, but having good sex is connected to women living longer.

Other studies on aging continue to point to connections between long life and sexual activity or satisfaction. In a study following more than 900 men over the course of ten years, they found that the risk of death was 50 percent lower among the men who had "high orgasmic frequency" of twice a week or more. Again, this does not mean that the orgasms were making them live longer, but the association between the two did remain when the analyses took into account other information about the men, such as their age, social class, smoking, and health status at the beginning of the study. There's evidence that sex helps older women stay healthy, too. For example, one study examined women who had difficulties or disabilities doing everyday tasks like bathing, dressing, or walking across a room. Among them, those who reported being satisfied with their sex lives were much less likely to develop a new disability. The older women who were more sexually satisfied were also staying healthier.

Of course, none of this is to say that there are not some real risks to your health from sex. Most notably, if you have unprotected sex and get infected with HIV or hepatitis, those infections will cut short your life. But for most people, good, frequent sex is connected to being healthy and living longer.

Squeezing Breasts Is
All Fun and Games

Squeezing breasts does sound like fun! When we look at the science, most women do love breast and nipple stimulation.

In one study assessing the role that the breasts or nipples play in sexual arousal, 81.5 percent of women reported that the stimulation of their nipples or breasts made them sexually aroused or enhanced their sexual arousal. And almost 80 percent of women said that, once they were aroused, having their breasts or nipples played with would increase their arousal even more. In fact, the majority of women had asked their partner to stimulate their breasts or nipples during sex.

Most men love it, too—not just playing with women's breasts, but also having their own nipples stimulated. At least half of men, 51.7 percent in one study, reported that stimulating their nipples would turn them on or enhance their arousal. But even if they like it, men are less likely to tell you that they want you to play with their nipples; only 17 percent reported that they had asked for this during sex in the past.

As fun as the breasts are, not everyone wants you to play with them. Among women, 7.2 percent report that manipulating their breasts or nipples will decrease their arousal. And a similar 7.5 percent of men find it to be a turn-off if you play with their nipples. Remember, you, too, can become a good researcher by experimenting with what your partner likes or does not like in this area.

Amazingly enough, there might be some benefits to breast squeezing that go beyond arousal and good feelings. Could squeezing breasts help fight cancer? This may seem like a teenage boy's wildest fantasy come true, but a lab at Berkeley has actually found that you can stop the malignant growth of a particular type of breast cancer cell with compression. They applied a very controlled type of squeezing or pressure to epithelial breast cancer cells and discovered that the pressure made them look less and less like messy cancer cells and more like normal cells. This "mechanical pressure" could halt the out-of-control growth of the cancer cells in comparison to the cancer cells that were left alone.

Now, no one has yet figured out if squeezing breasts can cure cancer. These studies were done with cells in a little dish in a laboratory, not with actual breasts. And we don't know if it would really improve the progression of the cancer long term, but it never hurts to have new ideas how to fight breast cancer. If you are looking for yet another reason to squeeze breasts—or to have your own squeezed—you can add this to your list.

Did we write this chapter just to talk about how great breasts and nipples are? Maybe, but it never hurts to add to your list of reasons to play with breasts.

Get Out of Those Pajamas!

Who thinks it is sexy to sleep in your pajamas? Comfort, thermoregulation, easy access . . . there are lots of good reasons to ditch the pajamas. Sleeping naked definitely seems sexy. Conversely, sleeping in pajamas seems much less so.

But if it's not sexy to sleep in your pajamas, very few people are taking the key step for sexy sleep. In a survey of over 3,700 Americans, only 8 percent reported that they sleep naked. Since 74 percent of the people surveyed reported that they sleep in pajamas that means plenty of sexy people must be sleeping in pajamas (or 74 percent of people are not sexy).

This was not a study of the highest quality. It did include a large number of people, but the survey was run by a company that makes linens (a company that is quick to point out that the naked minority might want to consider buying soft sheets). Nonetheless, even with the limitations of this survey, it is interesting to think about what people wear or do not wear when they sleep.

Men are more likely than women to embrace nude sleep. In a telephone survey of 1,501 adults in the United States that was conducted by ABC News, 31 percent of men reported sleeping in the nude, compared to 14 percent of women.

There may be some other health benefits to sleeping in the nude. Among a small group of patients with skin disorders, overheating during sleep was found to be an issue that made their skin disorders worse. (Losing your rash might also be sexier!)

Can't Buy Me Love

For many years, across many societies, the decision about whom to marry depended a great deal on money. Men with more wealth had their pick of eligible young women, and finding a wealthy husband was a high priority. In more recent years, in many parts of the world, it has become much more likely that your spouse will be chosen based on a wider range of factors that might include mutual interests, similar levels of education, and even love.

How money and sex are tied together remains an interesting question for those of us in places like North America and Europe. We often like to think that money does not have much to do with it, but other than the obvious transactions where people pay money for sex, are money and sex linked in today's world?

Two scientists who specialize in behavior and evolution, Daniel Nettle and Thomas Pollet, have reported that wealth still makes a difference for natural selection (meaning that money makes a difference in terms of who has babies). Looking at data collected for 5,575 men and women in Britain who were followed for over forty years, the researchers found that men with higher levels of income were more likely to have children, even taking into account differences in the level of education. While this link between having more money and having more children is seen across many cultures, it is much stronger in poorer countries than it is in wealthy countries like the United States and Britain.

It makes sense that men with more money might be seen as better options for being able to support a child, but what about the actual sex?

These same two researchers published a very controversial study that connects women's orgasms with their male partners' wealth. They surveyed Chinese men and women, and found that a woman's orgasms and a man's income tracked together. The more money a man was making, the more orgasms a woman reported. The researchers took into account a lot of other characteristics of the couples, including age, happiness, education level, how long they had been together, the differences in wealth or education between the partners, and which region they lived in. Separate from all of these other factors, money was connected to orgasms.

In trying to explain why this might be the case, the investigators speculated that men who make more money may demonstrate other things that women want—the ability to provide for children, good genes, high status. Having more orgasms could bond the women to these men—whether sexually or emotionally—and therefore increase the chance that they will have babies. On the other hand, wealthier men might also act different in bed. Richer men do report higher levels of self-esteem, and this could also impact their bedroom behavior, and how they have sex with a woman.

Another study, which surveyed 5,407 people in Chile across twenty-four cities, found that a high socioeconomic status was associated with higher levels of sexual satisfaction for women, but not for men. Education level and sexual satisfaction were also tied together for both women and men. However, in the analyses that put all of the potential information about the men and women into the equation, being in love with your partner was, by far, the best predictor of being satisfied sexually. Next came having a good sex life in the past, with having a high educational level coming in after that. The socioeconomic status, which represents your money and status, was not significant.

Before you start thinking that you better make a lot of money or no woman will want to sleep with you, you should know that not every study looking at women's sexual function shows that money makes a difference. In a smaller study, one that interviewed a random group of 436 women and their partners, there was only a very weak tie between having a higher socioeconomic status (meaning, more money and status) and how often they had orgasms or how much they enjoyed their sexual activity. Finally, in a much, much bigger study of almost 16,000 adults in the United States, income level was not tied at all to whether you had more or less sex.

Plus, it is possible that if you *are* having sex, that will make you just as happy as money. Among the 16,000 Americans, it was very clear that the more sex a person had, the happier they were. This was true for both men and women; having sex at least four times a week was associated with a big boost in happiness. (About half as much of a boost as being married, but it was still a big boost.) Having a higher income level also boosted happiness points, but how much money you made and how much sex you had did not interact with each other. Money bought the participants neither more sex nor more sex partners.

In these types of analyses, scientists actually try to calculate how happy one thing versus another thing will make you. They want to try to figure out what will maximize happiness. It turns out that the number of sex partners that one needs to maximize happiness is just one. This may go along with the fact that married people have much more sex than those who are single, divorced, widowed, or separated.

And while money does not seem to buy you any more sex by their estimates, it does seem that sex can buy you as much happiness as money can.

Television Makes You Oversexed

Television shows contain plenty of sex. An estimated 75 percent of prime-time television shows have something related to sex going on, and talking about sex is estimated to occur as many as eight to ten times in an hour of prime-time television. There isn't a lot of talk about safe sex, either; studies counting up the sex on television estimate only 14 percent of the sex content also includes some discussion or reference to the risks or responsibilities that go along with sex.

All of this sex on television makes some people very nervous about children and teenagers. There have been several studies that show an association between watching sexual stuff on television or other forms of media and starting to have sex earlier. The question remains open as to whether the sex on television is actually *causing* kids to start having sex earlier or whether kids who watch things with a lot of sex are also the same kids who start having sex earlier for other reasons.

The current research does offer suggestions that watching sexy stuff might push some adolescents to have sex earlier. Out of nine studies that followed almost 10,000 children over time, and examined both what kinds of media they were exposed to and when they started having sex, seven studies found that children exposed to more media and to more sex in the media were at a significantly higher risk of beginning to have sex earlier in life. In contrast, adolescents with parents who put limits on how much television they watched also waited longer to have sex. It's difficult to say whether this was actually because of the television or because the kids had stricter parents all around.

As much as we worry about television provoking this kind of rampant lust or sexual behavior, it seems to have a very different impact on adults. In fact, watching more television seems connected with having less sex!

In a survey of about 1,000 American adults, watching more television was tied to sleeping less and having poorer sleep habits, and these problems with sleep were then tied to negative effects on the adults' intimate and sexual relationships about 20 percent of the time.

Having a television in your bedroom might be particularly bad for your sex life. According to an Italian researcher who interviewed over 500 Italian couples, you might have sex twice as often if you were a couple without a television in your bedroom. The couples with televisions in their bedroom had sex an average of four times a month. In contrast, the couples without televisions in the bedroom averaged having sex eight times a month or twice a week.

One politician in India has gone as far as to suggest that television might serve in the effort for population control! In 2009, he was advocating that people in India should address the problem of overpopulation by watching more television and having less sex. We would note that there are much, much more effective forms of contraception than television. Oral contraceptive pills, condoms, and IUDs all come to mind. Nonetheless, you might think about whether your television is getting in the way of your sex life. It just might make you undersexed instead of oversexed.

It's Only a Matter of Time Until a Man Cheats

The seven-year itch, a popular meme in all kinds of media, refers to the belief that there is a time when men (and sometimes women) begin to wander in their marriages. In a broader sense, however, it refers to the belief that over time, people are more likely to want something outside of their relationship. Along these lines, many people believe that older men are more likely to have an affair.

This myth is reinforced by the idea of "trophy wives." Men may age, but they always want younger women. So an older man is more likely to abandon his older wife for a newer model.

But is this myth true? Are older men more likely to cheat?

Before we get into this, it's important for us to consider why this is important. Human beings in relationships can get caught between a number of competing feelings and instincts—jealousy, lust, a desire for passion, wanting to protect their partner or family. The idea of infidelity is a worrisome one for many people, and they want to know the warning signs for an affair. They want to know how to predict one.

A ton of research has looked at what factors might be related to infidelity.

Unfortunately, a lot of it is contradictory. Older work pointed to the fact that men were more likely to cheat than women. In recent years, though, that difference has dwindled. These differences also depend on what you define as cheating. If you require intercourse to call it an affair, men may do it more often. If you're willing to accept other acts as cheating, women are pretty much the same as men.

Religion can be a mediating factor. A number of studies have shown that people who endorse some sort of religious affiliation are less likely to report infidelity than those who do not. Of course, religion might change what people feel comfortable reporting more than it changes what they actually do.

Many believe that education and income can also predict infidelity. Some studies suggest people with more education and who make more money are more likely to engage in affairs. But it is not clear whether this is really due to education or money, or to the fact that people with these things have more opportunities to cheat. Is it the money, or the freedom it purchases?

But most of these factors are red herrings. They are an attempt for us to blame something external for the infidelity that we might see. When we focus on these factors, we can tell ourselves it's not something in the relationship—it's something in the person or their environment.

Does age make a difference?

One rigorous study published in 2011 in the *Archives of Sexual Behavior* looked at this question. The study evaluated 506 men and 412 women who were in reportedly monogamous sexual relationships. They examined a host of potential factors that might be associated with infidelity. Age did not turn out to be one of them. How can this be?

Well, part of the reason is how we ask the question. If you

are interested in whether a man has ever had an affair, then it is quite obvious that men who are older will be more likely to answer such a question positively. After all, older men have had more years in which they might cheat. As they age, the accumulated chance of cheating can only go up. But what we really want to know is at what age a man is most likely to cheat. And when it comes to that factor, age is not nearly as relevant.

What is? A host of factors. This comprehensive study found that about 23 percent of men and 19 percent of women had cheated during their current relationship. Most of the results are not surprising. People who are unhappy in their relationships and are somewhat incompatible in terms of sexual attitudes and values are more likely to stray. Such factors are far more important than demographic factors.

And in the end, that makes perfect sense. People who are unhappy, or who are mismatched in some way are more likely to cheat than those who are not.

So stop worrying about the age of your partner and start worrying about the quality of your marriage. Not only will that reduce the chance of infidelity, it will make your relationship better as well.

There's a Ten-Year Difference in Sexual Peaks

*M*en reach their sexual peak at eighteen, but women don't reach theirs until twenty-eight. We've heard this myth so many times, it's one we assumed must be true. But as with all myths, we still needed to prove whether it's so. But this is one of those myths that requires some extra thought before getting to work.

What does it mean to peak sexually? Does it mean the age at which you most want sex? Or is it the age where you are having the most sex? Is it the age when sex is the most satisfying? The most varied? Does any of this matter, or do all of these things happen at the same time?

A number of people believe that this myth originated with our local heroes, the researchers at The Kinsey Institute. The Kinsey Institute reports found that women have more orgasms in their thirties than at any other decade in their lives. This led many to postulate that women were having more satisfying sex then because they were more comfortable at this age, i.e., they were in their "sexual peak." Men, on the other hand, pretty much start orgasming during sex as soon as they have it.

Others think this myth might have a more scientific origination. Men's testosterone level peaks at around age eighteen, but women's estrogen levels peak in their mid-twenties. Since low hormone levels have been associated with lower sexual drive, some have asserted the opposite must be true. When your levels are at their highest, your drive must be at its peak.

But getting back to our original questions, what does it mean to peak? If we believe frequency of sex to be the factor that matters most, then both men and women are least likely to go without intercourse for a whole year during their late twenties. There's no difference between them. Single men are most likely to have sex four or more times a week in their thirties, and partnered men are most likely in their forties. For single and partnered women, such frequent sex is most likely in their late twenties. So if this is our metric, men are peaking after women.

Men and women are most likely to masturbate alone in their late twenties. Men are most likely to receive oral sex in their thirties and to give it in their late twenties. Women are most likely to receive and give oral sex in their late twenties. Men are most likely to have anal sex in their early twenties; women are most likely in their late twenties.

We're not trying to say that there's a pattern here. But it's pretty obvious that there's no magic number for men and women. Moreover, it's truly clear that men don't peak early and women late.

Common sense tells us that people's sexual drive is not on a constant trajectory throughout their lives. Do you think your sex drive goes up until it hits a high, and then declines steadily until you die? Not true. Sexual desire constantly fluctuates, and is related to many, many more factors than age. It's likely that over the course of a lifetime, you will see your sexual desire and activity go up and down many, many times. But one thing is for sure. Men need not worry that it's all downhill after eighteen, and women don't need to feel like they will always be out of sync with men. It's much more complicated than that.

Only Teenagers Come Too Soon

Although no one really likes to talk about it in public, most of us share a common vision of what premature ejaculation looks like. A man and a woman are inching closer and closer to sexual intercourse when suddenly the man loses control. The venue in which this occurs, the state of undress, the response of the participants—all these variables are up for grabs. But all of us imagined one thing similarly. The male participant is young. Most likely, he's a teenager.

There's a perception that premature ejaculation is a boy's problem. Full of hormones and out of control with desire, the young man is so excitable that he just can't wait. He's so eager and inexperienced that he cannot control himself, and he winds up orgasming at the completely wrong time. On this, we all seem to agree.

But is this perception correct? Is premature ejaculation a young man's problem? Or are we falling prey to another myth about sexuality?

Let's start with some basic facts about premature ejaculation. A number of studies have estimated the prevalence of sexual disorders. One particularly good one was published in *JAMA* (*The Journal of the American Medical Association*) in 1999. Researchers used data from the National Health and Social Life Survey, which included a random sample of almost 2,000 adults in the United States. They asked about a number of sexual dysfunctions that occurred in the last year, including "climaxing too early." They found that 30 percent of eighteen- to twenty-nine-year-olds reported this issue. But almost identical numbers of thirty- to thirty-nine-year-olds (32 percent), forty- to forty-nine-year-olds (28 percent), and fifty- to fifty-nine-year-olds (32 percent) reported the issue. It absolutely did not trend toward younger males.

For the vast majority of these men, premature ejaculation is a transient and temporary issue. Almost all recover from it and do not have it occur again. Others may require some reassurance, education, or behavioral therapy. Almost none need medical treatment, and almost none have it disturb their sex lives in a long-lasting way.

But experts will tell you that there are more serious types of premature ejaculation. Lifelong premature ejaculation is a chronic condition in some men where the problem occurs with nearly every woman and in nearly every episode of intercourse. Almost all men with this condition come less than a minute after inserting their penis into a vagina, and pretty much all do within two minutes. But here's the thing. For most of these men (70 percent), it's a lifelong problem. In fact, in more than a quarter of them, it gets worse as they get older. Unlike the temporary reports in the *JAMA* study, though, this problem likely afflicts less than a few percent of men.

Acquired premature ejaculation is a different issue altogether. In this form, the man starts to have problems with premature ejaculation at some point after he already had a history of normal ejaculation. This is most often due to some organic disease or condition that is interfering with normal sexual function. These conditions could include urologic issue, thyroid disease, or psychological issues. Almost all of these can be fixed with proper treatment of the underlying issue, and almost all of them are not likely to occur in younger men. In fact, many are more likely to occur in older men.

It's unlikely that the portrayal of males suffering from premature ejaculation will change in the media. There is, after all, a certain comedic value in depicting a hapless young boy losing control in a sexual encounter. But the next time you think of premature ejaculation, we hope that you will take a more realistic view of it. It can occur in men of any age. In fact, there are types that are far more likely to occur in older men, not younger. And because there are many things that can be done to treat the problem, we would suggest talking to your doctor if you think this is a problem for you or your partner.

Watching Porn Is a Guy Thing

In 2009, researchers in Montreal were trying to do a study of men in their twenties. They wanted to compare the view of men who had never watched pornography to those who regularly did. There was one problem. They couldn't find a single man who had never watched porn.

This was a small study, and these results were repeated for the most part only in the lay media, but they perpetuate two stereotypes: 1) all men watch porn, and 2) porn is a guy thing.

Let's start with the first question. How many men do watch porn? One of the most comprehensive studies around was just recently published, and used data from the General Social Survey, which is a massive national survey funded by the National Science Foundation that has been collecting data on social beliefs and behaviors of people in the United States since 1973. Researchers took a look at results from this survey from then until 2010. Over the nearly three decades, that included more than 14,000 males in the United States.

Now, before we look at the results, it's time for some truth. We totally believed that the results of the Montreal researchers would have been proven true writ large. Have you been on the Internet lately? Some days it seems impossible not to see porn. But we were willing to put aside our biases and look at the evidence.

We were shocked. In 2010, only 36 percent of men reported having watched at least one pornographic film in the last year.

In 1973, that number was 31 percent. With some minor fluctuations to a low of 20 percent in 1980 and a high of 30 percent in 1987, that number hasn't changed that much. Over all the years, the percent of men who responded affirmatively was about 32 percent.

When you look at these numbers, one thing you have to remember is that lots of men are older men. And the older you are, the less likely you are to watch pornography. Whites are slightly less likely to consume pornography than males in minority groups. And people who are more religious are slightly less likely to watch pornography as well.

This isn't to say that pornography isn't a huge business. Video pornography was generating more than $10 billion a year more than a decade ago. That number has only increased since then.

So are these low numbers even possible? Doesn't everyone watch porn?

It turns out the answer is no. In 2005, researchers reported that only 14 percent of people reported ever having explicitly visited a sexual Web site. We know that sounds hard to believe. You have to remember, though, that the Internet use skews young. It's likely your grandparents aren't trolling the Web for porn. Lots of people are in that age demographic. And even among younger people, it's not as frequent as conventional wisdom might have you believe. A 2007 study conducted by researchers in New Hampshire surveyed 1,500 Internet users between the ages of ten and seventeen years of age. They found that even in the oldest age range (sixteen to seventeen years old), less than 40 percent of boys were looking for pornography voluntarily.

But do females and males watch pornography in equal amounts? More women may see pornography than you think, but it still may be mostly a guy thing.

First of all, we have to acknowledge that almost all of the research seems to be on boys. Therefore, it's a bit of a self-fulfilling prophecy. But when studies do look at both sexes, differences seem to emerge. Among the sixteen- and seventeen-year-olds, while almost 40 percent of boys were seeking out pornography on the Internet, less than 10 percent of girls were. An additional 30 percent of boys were "accidentally" exposed to pornography, compared to about 38 percent of girls. So overall, boys sought out much more pornography than girls. Another study found that two times as many males were using sexually explicit Internet sites as women, and were spending more time on them as well. More than half of women, on the other hand, reported that they never downloaded sexual material at all.

Of course, they could be lying. But we tend to believe in the reliability of anonymous surveys, as research generally shows that they return truthful results.

Bottom line: Men do access pornography more than women, but pretty much everyone is viewing pornography much less than the media would have you believe.

Men Want It More. Way, Way More.

This is one of those myths so accepted as truth that it's hard to even muster the energy to fight it. You probably won't believe us anyway. You probably believe that men think about sex every seven seconds.

As we've discussed in previous books, that's not even possible. That would mean that men would have to think about sex more than 57,000 times a day, or pretty much every time they took a breath. That would not only drive most people mad, it would make them incapable of performing any other functions at all. Men are not being driven crazy with thoughts of sex every seven seconds.

But to be completely truthful to the data, men do think about sex more than women do. A very comprehensive study on the subject was published in 1994. More than half of men reported that they think about sex every day or several times a day, versus only 19 percent of women. Just over 40 percent of men reported thinking about sex a few times a month or a few times a week, versus 67 percent of women. Only 4 percent of men said they think about sex less than once a month, versus 14 percent of women. Yes, men think about sex more than women.

But this is a difference that's far less dramatic than you might otherwise think. Almost half of men don't think about sex every day. That's a far cry from the way they are often portrayed in the media. The myth of the sexually obsessed male is not accurate at all. Men think about many, many, many other things each day—far more than they think about sex.

Perhaps you are less interested in how many times men think about sex than how many times they actually have sex. If we stick to vaginal intercourse, the differences are much less than most would think as well. Let's take single people first. About 57 percent of men age eighteen to twenty-four have not had sex in the last year, versus 51 percent of women. You read that correctly. More women had sex than men. In fact, 5 percent of single women age eighteen to twenty-four had sex four or more times per week versus 2 percent of men. Single women have more sex than single men in the twenty-five to twenty-nine age group as well. Women finally start to fall behind men when they hit thirty—which is, of course, further proof that it's a myth that women peak sexually when they are older (see "There's a Ten-Year Difference in Sexual Peaks").

The numbers for married men and women are similar. Married women have more sex when they are eighteen to twenty-four; married men have more sex when they are twenty-five to twenty-nine. After that, the numbers are comparable.

None of this is to convince you that women have way more sexual urges than men, or that they act on them far more. We'd be happy splitting the difference. There's compelling evidence that there just isn't that much difference between men and women when it comes to sex. Men think about sex more, but may be less likely to actually have sex at many ages. And it's a myth to think that women don't want sex. We'd be thrilled if people would just show a little more equivocation and uncertainty about who has more or less sex or sexual thoughts.

You also need to remember that these are averages of large populations. There is little doubt that some men think about sex a lot. There's also little doubt that some men have a ton of sex. But that holds true for some women, too. The individual anecdote does not define the gender. Population level data shows this myth just isn't true.

I Can't Do That . . . It Will Give Me Hemorrhoids

Although it seems far more mainstream than it used to, anal sex is still one of those topics that seems most discussed in whispers and in private. It also has, in the past, carried somewhat of a taboo. One reason, obviously, is that it is not directly related to procreation. Another is that is has been attributed to homosexual males. But anal sex is not uncommon in the heterosexual population, though it still seems to be less openly discussed than other practices.

Because of this, many myths center around the activity. One of these is that anal sex causes hemorrhoids. Before we can even discuss the myth, though, it's important to understand exactly what hemorrhoids are.

There's no good way to put this: Hemorrhoids are swollen veins in your anus or lower rectum. Internal hemorrhoids are usually in the rectum and hidden, while external hemorrhoids are under the skin around the anus. Internal hemorrhoids are more likely to be painless. You won't notice them except by blood in your stool (which, of course, can cause you to panic). External hemorrhoids can cause pain, itching, and discomfort. They, too, can bleed.

Hemorrhoids are surprisingly common. About 50 percent of adults have had a case of hemorrhoids by the age of fifty. Since blood in your stool can be associated with a host of things far worse than hemorrhoids, it's always a good idea to get it evaluated when you see it. Hemorrhoids themselves rarely result in serious problems, except when the bleeding is really bad. Your doctor will make a diagnosis pretty much by looking for them, either seeing them around your anus or using a scope to look inside. But there's no other test or scan that is used to look for hemorrhoids.

Mild hemorrhoids are treated with topical medications, like creams, pads, or suppositories. These can often help with discomfort or itching. Sometimes, there are other noninvasive ways to treat them. Hemorrhoids can be "banded" with, of all things, rubber bands. By putting a small rubber band around the bottom of an internal hemorrhoid, it can be "strangled" of blood, and then it will fall off in a number of days to a week. (Do not try this at home!) Doctors can also inject medicine into hemorrhoids to shrink them, or use laser or infrared treatments to harden and shrink them. Less commonly, bad hemorrhoids may require surgery.

But let's get back to the original question. What causes hemorrhoids? Quite simply, it's from increased pressure in your lower abdomen. The more pressure you put there, the more blood floods into the veins and potentially causes a hemorrhoid. One common way this happens is by straining while making a bowel movement. In fact, this is the reason so many people tell you not to push when you're sitting on the toilet. The constant strain can lead to hemorrhoids. Another common cause in women is pregnancy. Having a baby in your belly adds quite a bit of pressure to your belly, and often results in hemorrhoids. Obese people are more likely to have hemorrhoids for this reason as well.

But all of these issues are chronic, meaning that they exist or build over a long period of time. Anal sex, on the other hand, does not. It's periodic, and unless you're shockingly out of the mainstream, your anal sex is not likely to occur continuously for months at a time, like a pregnancy would. You don't get hemorrhoids from rubbing or stretching the anus; you get hemorrhoids from increased pressure in the lower abdomen. It is pushing more blood into the veins that make hemorrhoids, not squeezing blood out of them.

It is possible, and even likely, that anal intercourse could exacerbate already existing hemorrhoids. It may even bring them to your attention, or make them symptomatic. Anal sex might make your hemorrhoids bleed or hurt. But that's not the same thing as causing hemorrhoids. Anal sex is unlikely to create a new hemorrhoid where none existed before.

As always, you should discuss concerns with your own physician. And remember that about 10 percent of both men and women report having had anal sex in the last year. You're not alone. Not even close.

You'll Never Go Gray . . . Down There

There are many things people don't look forward to when they age. One of those things is watching your hair turn gray. While you see it happening to the hair on your head, and even to your facial hair, you might find yourself taking comfort in knowing that your pubic hair will not change as you get older.

Or will it?

It's probably a good idea to start with an explanation of why hair turns gray in general. Hair grows from follicles in your skin at the base of each shaft of hair. Every follicle contains cells called melanocytes that produce a pigment known as melanin. The color of your hair is determined by how much melanin is in each strand of hair. It is the melanocytes that put that melanin into your hair and give it color.

Until they don't. As you get older, the melanocytes in your follicles begin to die. They aren't replaced. As they die, the hair coming from that follicle loses its color and starts to look gray. This usually takes many years.

We hope you noticed that the coloring of hair takes place in the follicle, at the base of each strand though. Once the hair leaves the follicle and grows, then the coloring is done. Hair can't change color radically once it's out of the follicle. Thus, stories you've heard of people whose hair has turned color overnight are just myths. The coloring takes place when the hair is formed, and is not changed after that.

But back to pubic hair. We hate to be the bearers of bad news, but the truth is that your pubic hair can turn gray just like all other hair on your body. People don't talk about it a lot, but it absolutely happens. We even found a study in the Japanese medical literature from 1995 where researchers used the amount of graying in pubic hair to estimate the age of men and women who were autopsied after death. Any elderly person with whom you can have a frank discussion about pubic hair will tell you the same thing: Pubic hair turns gray eventually.

The good news is that it may not happen right away. Even by the age of sixty-five, some men and women had no gray in their nether regions. But males might see gray hairs as early as thirty years old, and women as early as thirty-six.

What do people do about this? Some accept it gracefully, as a part of aging. Some choose to get rid of all their hair entirely, much as some men do on their heads or faces. But some choose to color their pubic hair just as they might their other hair. Do a search on the Internet, and you'll find any number of products to help you.

One word of caution though—do you remember the chapter on grooming your pubic hair (see "Bald Is Best") and the tens of thousands of injuries that people sustain each year because of grooming their pubic hair? You have to be very, very careful about using strong chemicals (such as hair dye) near your delicate bits.

Let's Play Back Door, Front Door, Back Door . . .

We want to be clear up front and say that this is not a chapter that is meant to scare you off of any kind of sex. All sex carries with it some form of risk, whether it be infection or pregnancy. As with everything, you need to weigh the benefits and harms of activities before you partake in them. For the vast majority of people, the benefits of most forms of sex outweigh the harms.

You can make the potential risks or harms of sex much less pronounced if you are careful. It is possible to protect yourself against an unwanted pregnancy. It's also possible to protect yourself against sexually transmitted infections. But still, there are sexual activities we engage in that are riskier than they need to be.

Anal sex, as we've discussed in a number of other chapters, is becoming more and more popular. In addition, it is becoming more and more popular to combine anal sex with other kinds of sex, like vaginal intercourse or oral sex. These combinations are rather common in pornography, and many people therefore assume that switching between anal and vaginal sex is safe.

There are real risks associated with putting a penis into the anus and then putting that same penis into the vagina. Gross as it may be to think about, the vagina has a host of normal bacteria inside of it that keep it healthy. (So does your mouth; so does your anus.) Taking something covered in the bacteria of the anus and rectum (which are basically poop bacteria) and then bringing those anal bacteria into the vagina can screw up (pardon the pun) the normal vaginal environment.

If you take a penis from the anus and put it in the vagina—even if it's covered by a condom—that penis will transmit bacteria from one place to the other. Plus, the moist, warm environment of the vagina is a nice place for bacteria to grow.

The introduction of new bacteria that don't belong in the vagina can throw off the normal healthy balance of bacteria in the vagina. An overgrowth of bad bacteria in the vagina is called "bacterial vaginosis," and it's not pleasant. It's the most common vaginal infection in women in the United States, especially in pregnant women. It can be accompanied by a discharge, a "fishy odor, pain, and itching." Women sometimes assume these symptoms are always from yeast infections, but this is different. Bacterial vaginosis can also increase your risk of getting another sexually transmitted infection. It can be treated rather easily with antibiotics, but it's important to do so as quickly as possible. This is especially true if you're pregnant, as it can be associated with bad outcomes for both the pregnancy and the unborn child. It's important to know that bacterial vaginosis is caused by other things besides anal sex, but it is a possibility when you go from having a penis in the anus to putting it in the vagina without cleaning the penis or changing condoms.

Don't take our word for it. A longitudinal cohort study of women published in 2008 followed 773 women for a year. One of the risk factors for bacterial vaginosis was "receptive anal sex before vaginal intercourse."

Your risk of other infections does not change much when you switch from anal sex to vaginal sex. If you already have HIV, for example, you can't get "more" HIV by spreading it from your anus to your vagina. HIV is an infection that is in your bloodstream, as well as in your semen or vaginal fluids. You could get HIV from anal sex or from vaginal sex, but once you have it, it is in your bloodstream either way.

Does this mean you need to abandon all thoughts of anal sex? No! But don't take the chance of creating infections. Be safe. If you're going to switch from anal sex to vaginal sex, change your condom. If you're not using a condom, which we don't recommend, then make sure to thoroughly clean anything coming out of the anus before it goes into the vagina. (This means soap and water, cleaning and drying.)

Another activity that is known to cause bacterial vaginosis, by the way, is douching. This is because douching also upsets the normal balance in the vagina, leaving women susceptible to the overgrowth of undesired bacteria. Don't do that, either. (Read all the reasons why you don't need to douche in order to be clean and fresh in that chapter!)

Married People Don't Play— with Themselves!

It's hard even to know where to begin with masturbation. Nearly everything we could say about it has been twisted into a myth. One such bit of information is the idea that married people might masturbate less. The idea is that people who have access to more ready sex have less reason to "take care of themselves." Is this true?

It's worth starting with some simple facts on masturbation itself. Good studies exist on the subject. One study of undergraduate college students found that 98 percent of males and 44 percent of females reported ever masturbating. The males averaged twelve times per month, and the women averaged five times per month. An older study, from 1994, found that about 60 percent of men and 40 percent of women said they had masturbated in the last year.

A much more comprehensive and recent study found similar results. Depending on their age, somewhere between 60 and 69 percent of men ages eighteen to fifty report having masturbated in the last month. For women, the range was 15 to 23 percent depending on age. Most men discovered masturbation between the ages of eleven and thirteen, but most women did later. And over their lives, only 5 percent of men and 11 percent of women never masturbated.

Bottom line: Nearly everyone has masturbated at one time or another. It's a very, very common and totally normal part of life.

Fewer studies look at how marriage might affect masturbation, but some do. One found that people living with a sexual partner masturbated more. About 85 percent of such men and 45 percent of such women had masturbated in the last year.

Why is this so? Well some more of the cynical-minded might say that married people get "bored" and are filling the void with masturbation. Others might say that married people are having less sex, and therefore they need to masturbate more. Of course, we've already disproven that myth—married people often have more sex than single people. Married people also have "better" sex in the sense that orgasm is likely to occur. Therefore, neither of these explanations seems likely.

It is more likely that married people are more comfortable with their sexuality over time. Because masturbation is often part of a healthy sexual life, married people who are more comfortable in their sexual lives might be more likely to masturbate as well. This is not a proven fact, but it is one possible explanation of the evidence.

What is fact is that married people do not masturbate less than single people. They have more sex, and they masturbate more.

Women Are Turned Off by Sweaty, Stinky Men

It seems like common sense that women would prefer their men not to smell. It seems obvious that after a workout, most women would prefer that their sexual partners take a shower and get cleaned up. After all, who would want a sweaty, stinky man?

It appears that women would.

In 2007, a group of scientists at the University of California, Berkeley, conducted a study of how certain components of male sweat affected women. They took a group of women and had them smell various compounds, one of which was androstadienone, a component of male sweat. They had them take twenty sniffs, and then give five saliva samples over a two-hour time period.

They found that women who smelled the androstadienone had had an improved mood and reported more sexual arousal. Those women also saw their blood pressure increase, their heart rates go up, and their breathing become more rapid.

What's more, those women also had higher levels of cortisol in their saliva. That hormone is part of the "flight or fight" response, and is often elevated in times of stress—including arousal. It is unclear whether the androstadienone caused the release of cortisol, which led to arousal, or whether the androstadienone caused arousal, which led to the release of cortisol. But what is known is that androstadienone leads to both mood changes and hormonal changes in women.

This work was novel in that it was the first time that a specific component of male sweat was found to influence women so specifically. It's also a subtle change. It's not like you can just whip up some androstadienone and see women lose their minds. This hasn't stopped some perfume and cologne manufacturers from including androstadienone in their scents.

Nonetheless, the next time you men have worked up a sweat, and are considering a shower before engaging that woman you're interested in, you may want to reconsider. That sweat may do more to help your case than hurt it.

When in Doubt, Double-Bag It

If one condom is good, surely two condoms are even better. Right? When it comes to "double-bagging," there are a few different things to consider. We are very much in favor of safe sex, but we want you to do it . . . safely!

A lot of people use more than one condom at the same time, at least in some parts of the world. In a study of the sexual experiences of 812 women in India, 485 had sex with a man using more than one condom at some point, and 39 percent had sex with a man using more than one condom at a time in the last month.

Maybe these women in India were trying to be extra safe, but many experts would tell them that using two condoms just makes them more likely to break. Obviously, this would make two condoms worse than one! These experts say that using two condoms at the same time creates friction between them that might result in one or both of the condoms tearing. This advice can be found on reputable health Web sites, and we have both heard doctors repeat this to patients, especially in the world of HIV prevention.

Just because doctors believe it does not make it true! Science does not support that using more than one condom at a time makes them break. Our searches of the medical literature did not turn up any studies at all that prove this point. The one study that we could locate comparing condom breakage rates suggests that breakage actually occurs *less* often when two condoms are used than when one is used.

In a study in Thailand, researchers examined 7,594 condoms used in 4,734 encounters between commercial sex workers and their clients. The condom breakage rate was 1.8 percent when just 1 condom was used, but it was 0.2 percent when 2 condoms were used. So, there was actually less breakage, which translates into better protection from sexually transmitted diseases and pregnancy.

On the other hand, there was also no real evidence that two condoms are better than one. In other words, the studies do not show any benefit to wearing two condoms, either; there is no evidence that two condoms better prevents the transmission of a sexually transmitted disease or pregnancy. One condom alone is plenty effective at both of these things.

Many men don't like wearing condoms, even though they are an amazing form of protection and birth control. It seems unlikely that those men would like wearing two more. If there's no benefit, we can't see the allure of putting on a second condom. Although if you wanted to go safely from anal sex to vaginal sex quickly, you could peel off that used condom and have at it.

Bottom line: One condom is a fantastic and safe way to have sex. Use it. If you want to use a second condom, feel free. There's no proof that it's safer, but there's also no proof that it's more likely to fail.

The Stiff Has a Stiff

Dead people having orgasms or erections? Some of these myths you don't want to touch. This is one of them. We wonder who even cares about this stuff. But evidently, there's a fairly large amount of media dedicated to this topic. Can dead men develop erections, and can they orgasm?

If you do an Internet search, you'll inevitably turn up a news story about a woman in Missouri who worked in a mortuary, and was arrested after becoming pregnant from a cadaver she, well, worked on. A little digging into the story, however, shows that it was originally published on a site known as Dead Serious News, which is a *satirical* Web site. It's not a real news source, and it's not a real story.

In fact, it's impossible for a cadaver to have an orgasm. In our first book, *Don't Swallow Your Gum!*, we explained that hair and fingernails do not keep growing once you have died because it takes a living body to undergo the complex hormonal regulation and physical action that results in true growth. The same is true of an ejaculation. A dead body is just that— dead. A cadaver is not producing sperm, it's not pushing fluids around, and it has no active nerves to know that stimulation is occurring.

But that's just orgasm. Can a dead body develop an erection? The key to answering this question is the word "develop." You see, if a cadaver doesn't have an erection at the time of death, one is not going to develop later. Again, there are no active nerves to know whether "arousal" is occurring. The blood that is necessary to pool to cause an erect penis doesn't flow after death. The muscles of a penis aren't working, either. The likelihood of a flaccid dead penis getting erect is about as likely as a dead corpse reacting to tickling or pain. It isn't going to happen.

But this doesn't mean that erections aren't found in dead bodies.

Depending on the means of death, it is possible for a body to die with an erection, and for that erection to remain. This is well documented in people who have died by hanging, and it is thought that pressure on the cerebellum causes some reaction. Interestingly, this does not appear to be limited to men. Women who have died by hanging can be found to have an enlarged or engorged clitoris and labia. Emissions, or ejaculations, accompanying the erections have been reported as well.

When a body dies with an erection, it may remain. Bodies harden after death and fluids congeal. If they do so in a state of priapism, a hardened penis may stick around after death. But that's a far cry from a cadaver developing an erection in response to stimulation, or an ejaculation occurring some time after death. That doesn't happen.

Did She or Didn't She?
Faking It for Beginners.

Although there are endless discussions of this topic to be found on the Internet, there's a surprisingly small amount of evidence proving whether you can spot the fake.

There's little doubt that most women have faked an orgasm at some time. The question is, of course, whether people can spot the fake. On this, there seems to be a great deal of debate.

Women believe that it's easy to spot a man faking it, as almost all men end an orgasm with some physical evidence. But a few men don't. (See the chapter, "There's Always Semen When You're Screamin.' ") Moreover, the use of condoms makes it much easier for a man to hide that evidence if he wants to.

Women, on the other hand, leave much less behind in terms of evidence. Female orgasms consist of physical movements, vocalizations, and attitude. All of those can be faked. While many, many articles can be found advising men on how to see through the acting, it's clear that a truly dedicated and talented woman could fool even the best of us.

Now that isn't to say we couldn't design a study to make this clearer. We could find a group of women and randomize them to fake it or not. Then we could pair them up with men and see if the men could tell who was acting. Of course, we'd have to make sure that the men were actually able to bring the women to orgasm. And we'd have to prevent orgasm in the fakers. And we're not really sure we could get any women to sign up for such a crazy study. Perhaps that is why no one has ever done a study like this.

There have been studies, though, where women underwent complicated brain scans and other monitoring in conditions where they were either being brought to orgasm, trying but not managing to get to orgasm, faking an orgasm, or at rest. These scans can detect a difference in brain activation and deactivation between these conditions. So, the scanner could tell a difference between a woman having a real orgasm and faking one—even if a man could not. This seems unlikely to help in practical situations.

A better question is *why* people fake orgasm. The most common reason reported is to make their partner happy. The second is because they want to get sex over with, and the third is because they don't want to hurt their partner's feelings. Few people report that they fake orgasm because the sex is bad.

In other words, most of the time, the reasons for faking an orgasm are somewhat altruistic. They are done to please someone else or spare their feelings. They're not faked because people are unhappy, or because they dislike or disdain their partner. If that's the case, why are we so eager to make trouble? We are all for having real orgasms, but sometimes it may be better not to be able to tell the difference.

Only Men Have Wet Dreams

Wet dreams, or an orgasm while asleep, are very common. More than 80 percent of men report them at some time in their lives. There have been a number of studies looking at what age wet dreams first occur, with results ranging from eight to twenty-six years. But all of these studies have been in boys. Because these studies are usually in boys, most people only think about nocturnal emissions (when a male ejaculates during sleep) as the only form of wet dreams that occurs.

But this is not the case.

Sex researchers usually define a wet dream as sexual arousal while asleep that culminates in an orgasm, which awakened them. As far back as the 1950s, Alfred Kinsey reported that almost 40 percent of the women he interviewed reported having a wet dream. A more comprehensive study was published in 1986 in the *Journal of Sex Research*. The author evaluated 245 women who were students at a large Midwestern university, and found that 37 percent of them said that they had experienced a wet dream. Moreover, 30 percent of them had had one in the last year.

We get why this myth might take root. After all, the evidence of an orgasm is much clearer in boys than in girls. Additionally, studies show that wet dreams are still viewed as something embarrassing in a number of cultures. Girls, as well as boys, might not want to talk about them. Since they are more likely to have plausible deniability, fewer may come forward to discuss them publicly.

It does seem that men are more likely to have a wet dream than women. No one knows whether this is the case, although lots of theories abound. We stick to science, though, and try not to create new myths through speculation.

What is indisputable is that women do experience wet dreams; they are not just confined to men.

Masturbation Will Make You Go Blind

People spend way too much time worrying about masturbation. There are so many ways people think it could hurt you. Masturbation will make you grow hair on your palms. Masturbating too much will make you go crazy. Masturbation will make you impotent later in life. Masturbation will make your penis curved. Masturbation will make you unable to have orgasms during regular sex. You shouldn't need to masturbate if you are in a relationship with another person. Masturbation will take away your virginity. Masturbation will sap your strength. All of these ideas are myths!

The evidence that masturbation will not make you blind or make hair grow on your palms is overwhelming. Lots and lots of people masturbate. In fact, even back in the 1940s, 94 percent of males and 40 percent of females reported having masturbated to orgasm. These numbers have only increased, with the percentage of females reporting that they have masturbated at 70 percent or more. In one study in the United States, half of American women reported using a vibrator. It is normal to masturbate.

And yet, while lots and lots of people are masturbating, not many people in the world are blind. Even fewer people grow hair on their palms. While mental illness is a real and common problem, it has no connection with masturbation. If masturbation really caused any of these problems, you would see lots and lots of blind, hairy, crazy people all around you. It just does not happen.

Even people who masturbate more often do not have physical problems from their masturbation. Researchers have looked closely at people who masturbated an average of four or more times a day over the course of years, and they were not any more likely to have any diseases than the people who masturbated less often. As we discussed in a previous chapter, masturbating won't make you run out of sperm, either. People who masturbate do not need to worry about their performance in sports or other feats of strength. Having sex or masturbating does not change how well you do on a treadmill and does not seem to change your strength, balance, reaction time, or aerobic power.

Masturbation is not going to deform your penis, either. Many men have curved penises or penises that are not perfectly straight. This is completely normal and has nothing to do with whether or not they masturbate. It should not have any negative impact on their experience of sex although we would recommend talking with a doctor if you have a specific concern about any part of your anatomy.

Masturbation can be a perfectly normal, healthy practice whether you are in a relationship or not. Giving yourself sexual pleasure can be an important way to practice sex, and it is probably the safest form of sex. Knowing what gives you pleasure can also lead to experiencing more pleasure with your partner. Masturbating should not ruin you for sex with another person. It can be a good alternative to sex with someone else, or it can be a healthy way to supplement your sexual relationship with your partner.

Sex Can Give You a Heart Attack

Once a person has had a heart attack, they often worry about whether or not they will be able to have sex again. Everyone has heard horror stories of people dying of a heart attack in the middle of sex, and those with a history of heart disease may be particularly afraid that sex is going to be too much for their heart. People seem to believe that various sexual antics are particularly strenuous for their heart. Please consult with a physician before boarding this ride!

But rest easy: Sex is not bad for your heart. In fact, having sex more often is connected to having a healthier heart. In a study that followed 1,165 men for an average of sixteen years, the men who reported having sex twice a week or more had a lower risk of developing cardiovascular disease. In contrast, men who engaged in sexual activity once a month or less had an increased risk of developing such disease during the study. The men who had sex less were 45 percent more likely to develop these heart-related problems, and this was unrelated to age or having a problem with erectile dysfunction. Whether having sex more often was a marker for being in good shape overall or whether it was tied to having a strong intimate relationship, having sex was strongly tied to having a healthy heart.

The chance of having a heart attack while you are having sex is also very low. A large study called the Framingham Heart Study has given us good information on these kind of risks by following lots and lots of men since 1948 and looking at their risk factors and heart problems. This study tells us that, if you are a man who does not have diabetes and does not smoke, the chance that you will have a heart attack during sex is one in a million! Even if you have heart disease, if you are able to pass a basic stress test, the chance you will have a heart attack during sex only goes up to ten in a million. From another study that looked at the determinants of heart attacks, we have learned that a fifty-year-old man who does not have heart disease and who has an annual risk of 1 percent for having a heart attack will only increase his risk of a heart attack to 1.01 percent if he has sex once a week. In case the numbers are confusing for you, the summary is this: The chance that you will have a heart attack during sex is quite low.

What if your heart has already had problems? One of the big concerns people have about having sex after a heart attack is that it will be too strenuous on their heart. While people who have had a heart attack do need to exercise some caution in terms of resuming normal activities, they do not need to be so afraid of having sex. The truth is that most people just do not exert themselves that much during sex! The physical exertion most people put in when having sex is similar to walking up two flights of stairs; sex does require some exertion, but it is not like running a marathon. Walking at about four miles per hour on a treadmill—the kind of stress test that heart attack victims will usually have to complete before they leave the hospital—is about the same level of exertion that you would have during sex that produces an orgasm. If you can do the treadmill walking, you are probably ready for sex. While a person who has had a heart attack usually needs to be careful about building up to their previous level of exercise, you will probably be ready for sex much sooner than for other activities. How soon you can resume sex also depends on what you mean by sex. Some sexual activities are more strenuous than others. The best way to know what you should or should not do and how soon you can do it is to talk with your doctor about your individual heart condition and what you would like to do sexually. Patients with particular symptoms or on certain drugs may need to be more careful than others, but your doctor can help you determine what your own risk level is.

Moreover, fear itself may be your biggest problem with having sex after a heart attack. If you are too afraid to have sex because you are afraid it will hurt you or your partner's heart, that fear could become the barrier to having healthy, enjoyable sex after a heart attack. This is another reason to talk with your doctor, and your partner, about the real risks involved, but also about the ways in which you can engage in and foster the loving, caring aspects of your sexual relationship.

Part Four

GETTING PREGNANT

You Can't Get Pregnant During Your Period

For most women, the chance of getting pregnant during your period is much less than at other times of the month. But it is never, ever impossible. Any time you hear someone say, "You can't get pregnant if . . ." you should think to yourself that someone is kidding themselves. If there is even a remote chance that a sperm and an egg are coming in contact with each other, then you can have a pregnancy.

It is much less likely that you will get pregnant during your period than during the time of the month a little before your period when your body sends an egg out, also known as the time when you are ovulating. Even though it is much less likely, it is still possible. The usual pattern of things is that a woman's body releases an egg, which travels through the fallopian tubes, which is where it would need to be fertilized by a sperm if she is going to become pregnant, and then the egg moves into her uterus and disintegrates if it has not been fertilized. Ovulation or the release of the egg usually happens two weeks before she starts her period. This is the time when pregnancy is most likely to occur.

If you have short menstrual cycles or irregular periods, there is a greater chance that you might have an egg present during the time that you are having a period. A woman's egg can live for several days, and not all women ovulate two weeks before their period. Some ovulate much closer to the time that the period occurs. Plus, sperm can live for days, even up to a week, in the nice, wet environment inside a woman's body. So, the combination of the egg being around and the sperm being around could lead to a pregnancy, even if the timing is unusual.

Some people attempt to use the "rhythm method" to prevent pregnancy. In other words, they only have sex during the "safe" days of pregnancy, when the woman is least likely to have an egg around. If you have really regular periods, you keep track of them carefully, and you can estimate the time when you ovulate by changes in the thickness of cervical mucus or body temperature, you might have a slightly better chance to avoid pregnancy for a while.

The rhythm method teaches us that no time is completely "safe" for avoiding pregnancy. Even when you are really careful about only having sex at "safe" times, the rhythm method is not a very effective method for preventing pregnancy. Timing your sex leads to pregnancies more often than using birth control pills, condoms, or injectable hormones. If you have sex without any of these other kinds of birth control, there is really no safe time to have sex.

If you don't want to get pregnant, use real birth control. And if you don't want to get a sexually transmitted disease, you need to use a condom.

If a Woman Has an Orgasm, It Is More Likely She Will Get Pregnant

For hundreds of years, men and women have had the idea that a woman is more likely to conceive if she has an orgasm during sex. Supposedly, in the 1600s in London, making sure that a woman did not have an orgasm during sex was a popular method of contraception (one can only imagine how this belief would play out in the course of a man and woman's relationship).

The theory, which has been described through various studies and physician investigations over the years, is that an orgasm causes the uterus to contract, which then creates suction through the cervix that would help semen to be sucked inside to where the sperms have a better shot at fertilizing an egg. This idea is often referred to as "upsuck."

Where this idea came from originally is not entirely clear; in the 1600s and 1700s, people had lots of crazy ideas about women's sexuality (as many still do today). Most of the scientific evidence for "upsuck" points back to a description published by a physician examining a single patient back in 1874. This woman had a prolapsed uterus, which means that her uterus had dropped down through the vagina, and her cervix at the bottom of the uterus was actually sticking outside of her body where it could be seen. The physician discovered that if the woman's clitoris was stimulated in a sexually arousing way, then he could observe the opening and closing of the cervix. This was used as proof that the cervix could actually be sucking in semen during orgasm. Since that time, quite a number of experts have criticized the scientific basis of this study—if you could even call it such. Most researchers would say that, since it only included one patient, it was not really a study. It included no other comparison patients and did not look at whether this movement had any impact on conception.

Since then, a number of studies have looked in more detail at how sperm travel through a woman's reproductive track. This is actually a very complicated process. When a man ejaculates, the sperm are released into the upper portion of the vagina through several spurts of ejaculate. The fluids mixed with the sperm actually contain different substances, depending on whether it is the first spurt or the last one. These fluids and chemicals combined with the sperm serve particular roles in allowing the sperm to survive in the vagina, to go through a process of "decoagulation" or unsticking that is necessary for them to be active, to help the sperm on their way in through the cervix and up through the uterus, and then to activate them for fertilizing that egg once they finally get to the fallopian tubes.

One of the interesting things about these studies of how sperm travel is that they usually look at the anatomy and mechanics of how the sperm make their way through the system, but they don't take into account what would happen if the woman is actually aroused. In other words, they don't look at the real life situation where arousal and orgasm creates changes in a woman's system.

During arousal, there are changes in the shape of the woman's vagina called "vaginal tenting." Once a woman is aroused, and before she has an orgasm, the vagina actually dilates or enlarges, which creates a sort of receptacle for the sperm to land in. The uterus does begin to contract when the woman has an orgasm, but the impact of these contractions is not known. They typically only last for a few seconds. Obviously, any "upsuck" would only be helpful if the sperm were already there, meaning if the woman is having an orgasm after the man has already ejaculated inside of her. We don't know whether "upsuck" of the sperm actually occurs. And even if it does occur, we don't know whether that difference in the woman's uterus helping to suck up the sperm more quickly actually results in more pregnancies compared to situations when the sperm are traveling up through the cervix without anything else going on. We really don't know if it makes a difference.

Studies have examined whether a chemical called oxytocin, which makes the uterus contract, could impact how fast dyes traveled up and into the uterus. Oxytocin did not make any difference in how fast the dyes were transported. Of course, there might be differences between the contractions from receiving doses of oxytocin as a medicine and the contractions that occur during an orgasm or when the body releases its own oxytocin.

We have clear proof, though, that women can become pregnant when all of this happens without an orgasm. In artificial insemination, we have many examples proving that sperm can be placed inside the woman's vagina in a clinical setting, and women can become pregnant even without any orgasms occurring.

In summary, we really don't know whether the contractions

of the uterus during orgasm play a role in moving sperm up into the uterus. When experts compile all of the most recent studies, they say that the current science suggests that orgasms do not impact the travel of sperm. There is no science to support that the way the uterus contracts during orgasm will increase the chance that a woman will get pregnant.

All these things being equal, there is no reason to believe that orgasms help for pregnancy. Women can certainly get pregnant without orgasms. Of course, the whole process of having sex is generally a lot more fun when everyone involved has an orgasm. So feel free to have one!

You Can't Get Pregnant
If It Was a Rape

In a perfect world, we wouldn't even have to include this chapter in the book. But even when we were writing it, this myth was still making the rounds. It even figured prominently in the 2012 elections, when former U.S. Representative Todd Akin made news by stating all too publicly that pregnancy from "legitimate rape" is rare. He went on to say that doctors had told him that women who were raped were traumatized in such a way that their bodies "shut down" the "whole thing" so that fertilization would not occur. He argued that this was a biological process.

As always, we start with the basics. The human body, like all of life on Earth, is about as efficient as it can be in making procreation possible. Many might make the argument that it's our primary purpose. Biologically, we're evolutionarily optimized to make it easier, not harder, for a woman to get pregnant. Women can get pregnant in all kinds of situations, even when they don't mean to. They can get pregnant if they have sex under water. They can get pregnant if they have sex during their periods. They can get pregnant almost any time of the month, in fact. If you put a sperm anywhere near an egg, it's possible for fertilization to occur.

We're not even sure what the difference is between "legitimate" and "illegitimate" rape. But that's a philosophical debate. To the female body, pregnancy happens when an individual sperm hits an individual egg. It doesn't matter how, or when, or why. The uterus doesn't know, and doesn't care, if it's from rape or not. Every year, there are many, many girls and women who get pregnant when they don't plan on it. No matter how much they wish it away, no matter how much they might not want to have a baby, they get pregnant. You can't control it with your mind.

Moreover, we've got epidemiological proof. More than 31,000 pregnancies from rape occur every year in the United States. Unless you want to start accusing them of "wanting" it, you can't actually believe that this myth is true. If so, you're declaring that every time a woman does get pregnant, she wanted it in some way.

That's a pretty horrible path to start down. It's much better to accept the scientific fact that will or desire or state of mind has nothing to do with biological fertilization, and just stop talking.

The Pill Will Make You Fat

Nearly all medications have side effects. When you are deciding whether a drug is right for you, it's entirely rational to weigh the potential benefits against the potential harms. But if one of those two things is a myth, then you might be making a foolish decision. For instance, many women forego one of the most effective methods of birth control—the pill—because they believe it causes weight gain.

Sadly, that's a myth.

It wasn't always the case. When the pill was first developed, it contained very, very high levels of both estrogen and progestin. These hormones, when taken correctly, prevent ovulation. Therefore, eggs don't leave the ovaries. Pills also cause cervical mucus to thicken, which can help prevent sperm from ever getting to eggs. Estrogen can cause increased weight gain in women, as well as water retention. Because of that estrogen, these original pills might have caused weight gain. But the pill as it exists today is much more refined, and contains far lower levels of hormones.

There is amazing science to tell us that today's birth control pills will not make you gain weight. Not only has the potential effect of contraceptives on weight gain been studied extensively, it has been studied so extensively that a meta-analysis, or study of studies, has been performed by the Cochrane Collaboration. They found forty-nine (yes, 49) studies that compared the pill to a placebo or other pills with respect to weight gain.

Four of the studies compared the pill to a placebo. None of them showed that birth control pills caused weight gain. Some studies that looked at different combinations of components in the pill, and most of these showed no relationship to weight gain, either. The studies also looked at whether contraceptives were stopped because of weight gain in the different groups, and once again—there was no difference.

Another systematic review (another study of studies) looked specifically at the influence of the pill on weight gain, among other factors, in girls younger than eighteen years of age. They found no evidence that the pill caused weight gain in adolescents. The combined study also found that obese girls didn't gain weight from the pill, either.

Since it's impossible to prove a negative, it's *possible* that some women will experience a very small amount of weight gain with the pill. After all, the pill does contain some estrogen. But these studies show that a measurable weight gain is very, very unlikely. In fact, it's much more likely that there is no relationship between the pill and weight gain at all.

This doesn't mean that birth control pills cannot have some serious side effects. They are often contraindicated if you have a history of breast cancer, lupus, heart or liver disease, or some other issues. You need a prescription to get the pill, and it's something you should discuss thoroughly with your doctor. But the upside is that the pill, when used correctly, is up to 99.9 percent effective in preventing pregnancy! Even if you forget a pill, it can still be 90 percent effective.

Most women can safely take the pill, and the large benefits usually outweigh the minimal risks. They especially outweigh the mythical risks like weight gain.

Birth Control Pills Don't Work as Well If You're on Antibiotics

Birth control pills are a pretty good method of birth control. They're not perfect; short of abstinence, nothing is. But there is a widespread belief that birth control pills will not work as well if you take an antibiotic at the same time. Some people suggest using condoms or some other additional method of contraception to protect against pregnancy if you need to be on an antibiotic.

Despite the frequent fears about this, and the warning labels you may see on some prescriptions, no good science exists to suggest that birth control pills don't work as well while taking antibiotics. One review by the American Academy of Family Physicians concludes that, while there are not a lot of good studies to help us answer the question, the scientific literature does not suggest that common antibiotics reduce how well birth control pills work. Some birth control pills have a low dose of the hormone to prevent pregnancy, and some of these might work less well when combined with antibiotics; but again, these decreases are very small. Another study looked at 356 patients in three dermatology practices with a history of long-term use of antibiotics and birth control pills together. There was no statistically significant difference between how many women got pregnant in the group on both antibiotics and birth control pills, and the control groups where women were on just the birth control pill.

Remember, birth control pills fail at least 1 percent of the time even in ideal conditions. And in studies that look at what happens in real life when women take an antibiotic with their birth control pill, the rate of getting pregnant doesn't seem to change.

Some science does suggest a theoretical possibility that one antibiotic, rifampin, might have the ability to make birth control pills less effective. In a study of thirty women that looked at the levels of drug in their blood, the level of the hormone in the birth control pill that prevents you from ovulating was lower when rifampin was used. None of these women got pregnant in the study, but the possibility was there. Rifampin is not an antibiotic that most women are going to encounter. It is usually used for tuberculosis or sometimes for meningitis.

Of course, future research with new drugs or more rare antibiotics might still mess up your birth control pills, but the science right now suggests that this is rarely a problem. It is much more important to take the pills every day and at the same time every day than to worry about most antibiotics. Look, there is no harm to wearing a condom if you want to be extra careful. But, you should not stop taking your antibiotic just because you are worried it will affect your birth control pills.

If You Put on the Pounds, Birth Control Pills Won't Work

To be honest, Aaron was unaware of this myth. But it didn't take much looking around to see that it's pervasive, especially among women. There is a widespread belief that the pill is less effective in obese or overweight women; it is even believed by healthcare professionals.

There's a logical reason for this. The pill is made up of a carefully calculated dose of hormones. These hormones interfere with a woman's fertility cycle primarily to prevent ovulation. This dose, like most drugs, was originally calculated by weight. Therefore, the dose a small woman receives is higher per kilo than what a large woman receives.

In fact, it seems counterintuitive that there shouldn't be larger pills for larger women. We must be overdosing tiny women or underdosing obese ones.

Some evidence supported this concern. In a study published in 2002 in *Obstetrics & Gynecology*, researchers reviewed the charts of 755 women followed at various times from 1990 to 1994. Of these, 618 used birth control pills at some time. During the study period, 106 pregnancies occurred. Most concerning, women in the highest weight quartile (above 155 pounds) had an increased risk of their birth control failing. The study also found that very-low-dose and low-dose pills were even more likely to be associated with failure.

As you can imagine, this caused a lot of consternation. These days, 155 pounds isn't even that high a weight in the

United States. Many women began to panic that their birth control would not work.

But retrospective studies like this can be flawed. They can be subject to recall bias. In other words, people who got pregnant may remember how they took their pills differently. They also can't prove causality. What would be more powerful are prospective studies that follow women over time. Those are usually more accurate.

One such study was published in 2009, in the *American Journal of Obstetrics & Gynecology*. They followed more than 59,000 users of birth control pills prospectively to see how various factors were related to failure rates. They found that failure rates were related to age (older women had fewer failures) and length of use (the longer the better). But both weight and BMI were unrelated to pill failure.

An even more powerful study was published in 2010. It was a randomized, controlled trial of two different doses of pills in both normal weight and obese women. The women didn't know which dose they were getting. The study was completed by ninety-six normal women and fifty-four obese women. Moreover, this study didn't use pregnancy as an end result. It actually measured ovulation through lab tests and transvaginal ultrasonography. Only four of the women ovulated during the study, and three of them were normal weight. In other words, there was no difference in failure rate between normal weight and obese women.

Finally, in 2011, the Cochrane Collaboration published a meta-analysis of studies on this subject. There were forty-nine of them. Some followed women on the pill as they gained or lost weight. Some were controlled trials of different pills or placebos. The bottom line was that there was no effect seen. Weight didn't seem to make a difference in whether the pill failed or not.

Of course, there are plenty of other reasons for women who are overweight or obese to try to get to a healthier weight. Pill failure just isn't one of them.

IUDs Are Horrible!

If you have ever considered your options for avoiding pregnancy, you may have heard some scary things about certain methods. For instance, there are many myths about intrauterine devices or IUDs. That's partly because you don't hear about IUDs in books, movies, television, and other media the way that you hear about condoms or the pill.

But IUDs are not uncommon. About 170 million women use them worldwide, making them the most common form of reversible contraception. They are the birth control of choice for more than 15 percent of all women who are married or living with a partner. They are also extremely effective. They have a failure rate of about 1 per 100 users in the first year and 3 per 100 users after five years. This makes them about the least likely to fail of almost any methods of contraception.

There are a number of different kinds of IUDs. Some are completely inert, and are just a foreign body in the uterus. Others contain copper, which has local effects in the cervical region. Some also contain progestogen, and release it slowly over time. All of them, though, work to decrease sperm motility and ability to survive long enough to make it to an unfertilized egg.

IUDs are abortion-causing contraptions!

What they don't do is cause abortions. Some people believe that all an IUD does is cause a fertilized egg to die. That's not the case. A study published in 1985 monitored daily blood samples in women over a fifteen-month period to see if they ever showed any signs of pregnancy. Three groups of women were followed: 1) women with IUDs, 2) women trying to get pregnant, and 3) women who had their tubes tied. The only women who ever showed the hormonal surge consistent with fertilization were in the group trying to get pregnant. Another study published in the same year used an even more sensitive laboratory test to look for a hormonal surge consistent in pregnancy. It found that in only 1 percent of 100 cycles in IUD users did fertilization occur.

Pregnancies do occur in IUD users, as they are not perfect in use in real life. The evidence is overwhelming, however, that they work by preventing fertilization, not by killing a fertilized egg.

IUDs cause infections in your uterus.

This is a modern myth that gained a lot of traction because it used to be true. There is a long and rich history of studies showing that the insertion of an IUD is associated with a significantly increased risk of a pelvic infection. IUD might have stood for Infectious Uterine Device! Almost all such research showed a really high rate of infection in the month following the placement of the device, and then a decrease in its incidence over time. This concern culminated in the United States with the furor over the Dalkon Shield. These IUDs had a tail made up of filaments encased in plastic that aided in its removal. Unfortunately, this plastic was found to crack over time inside the woman's vagina or uterus, exposing the filaments to the rest of the world. Bacteria could colonize in these filaments, which then climbed up into the pelvic area, causing an infection.

When it comes to new IUDs, we don't have the same worries. More modern devices and studies in more recent years do not appear to show these same rates of infection. They are sometimes higher than we'd like to see, but not nearly as high as in the past. But even those slight differences have been called into question. This is partly a fault with how the studies themselves are designed and conducted. Many of the studies were conducted in other countries in ways which make them difficult to generalize to the United States.

But a larger concern is what the IUD is being compared to. You see, other contraceptives, like condoms or ointments, can actively work to reduce the rates of pelvic infections. So when you compare the IUD, which does not prevent infection, to them the IUD looks much worse. But this doesn't mean that the IUD is causing infection. It's just that IUDs don't prevent them. A better-designed study would compare the IUD to no contraception at all.

When all of this is put together, it appears that the rates of infection in IUD users today don't seem to be much different from those of sexually active women who don't use them. In other words, they don't cause infections.

You are not going to be able to have children if you use an IUD.

Almost no debate about the use of IUDs is as heated as this one. It stems from two papers that appeared in *The New En-*

gland Journal of Medicine in the mid-1980s. Both of them concerned women who had never been pregnant before. The first found that compared to women who had never used an IUD, a woman who had ever used one had a 260 percent chance of developing primary tubal infertility. The second study found similar results, especially for the Dalkon Shield, which increased the risk 330 percent over never having used an IUD. However, even in those studies, women who had used the IUD with only a single partner saw no increased risk or infertility.

Immediately, IUD use massively decreased in young women who had never been pregnant. But research that followed began to contradict the earlier findings. A study out of Norway in 1988 showed that 100 percent of the women in the study were able to get pregnant within thirty-nine months of stopping IUD use. Some people theorized that perhaps women who had their IUDs removed because of complications would be more likely to develop infertility. The Norway study did not include such women. So a study out of New Zealand, following up data on more than 1,050 women who had used and then had IUDs removed for any reason, looked at this question. They found that there were no significant reductions in fertility for women who had complications than in those who didn't.

These days, the overwhelming evidence shows that the risk of significant pelvic infection from having multiple partners is the true cause of increased rates of infertility. Monogamous women who use IUDs have no real risk for infertility. This was made explicit in a 2001 study in Mexico, that proved that it is pelvic infections, and not IUD use, that is associated with infertility. If you want to stay fertile, don't worry about IUDs; worry about infection from having multiple sexual partners.

IUDs cause significant bleeding or pain.

One of the reasons women cite for not wanting to use IUDs are a concern that they cause significant bleeding or pain. One study showed that about one in five women who use copper IUDs report heavy bleeding for the first three months, but that seems to go away over time. Another larger study found that menstrual flow increased in about 30 percent of copper IUD users, but that hemoglobin level stabilized before a year of use.

It is true that these complaints are cited by some women who choose to have their IUD removed. But it's important to put this concern in context by comparing it to other forms of birth control. It turns out that women who use IUDs are much more likely to continue using them than other forms of birth control. A study in France found that women who use an IUD do so continuously for an average of fifty-five months. Women who use the pill, though, do so continuously for only forty-three months. They use condoms continuously for nineteen months, and spermicides continuously for thirteen months.

So women who use IUDs use them for a relatively long time. If these bleeding concerns were really so overwhelming, it's likely that more women would abandon the IUD as a method of birth control. That doesn't happen.

Want a Baby Girl? Turn This Way, Bend That Way.

Aaron's first two children were boys. By the time he and his wife were trying for a third child, many, many discussions occurred about how to influence the sex of their next child. (Spoiler: His third was a girl). One thing people believe might make one gender or the other more likely is the position in which a woman is impregnated.

First of all, if it were possible for this to work, everyone would know. Everyone. Not only that, everyone would be getting only the gender they wanted in children. Obviously, this doesn't happen. Why? Because you can't influence the gender of a fetus in this fashion.

The sex of a baby is solely determined by the sperm of the father. Period. Every single egg in a woman's body contains an X chromosome. Sperm, on the other hand, come with X and Y chromosomes. If the X chromosome fertilizes the egg, it's a girl. If a Y chromosome fertilizes the egg, it's a boy. That's how it works.

We've heard some pretty incredible stories as to how this might be affected by sexual position. One version has it that X sperm are bigger than Y sperm, because the X chromosome is significantly bigger than the Y chromosome. Therefore, if ejaculation occurs further from the cervix, Y sperm have a better chance of overtaking X sperm and making it to the egg first. So if you want a girl, go for a deep ejaculation. If you want a boy, do the opposite.

Of course, chromosomes are really, really small, and the difference between the weight (and the speed) of X and Y sperm is negligible. Also, sperm don't swim in a direct line. They are just as likely to start swimming in the wrong direction as the correct one. So it's not a 100-meter dash where the faster sperm is always going to win.

Another explanation has it that X sperm are hardier than Y sperm. So if you ejaculate farther from the cervix, X sperm are more likely to make it to the egg first. Did you note that this is the exact opposite advice? If this is true, if you want a boy, go for a deep ejaculation. If you want a girl, do the opposite.

Again, though, if this were the case, then there would be many more women than men in the world. X sperm would be more likely in general to live long enough to make it to the egg. That's not the case. It's pretty much a 50/50 chance. Always.

The truth? Both of these things are true to some extent. Y sperm are slightly faster and X sperm are slightly more hardy. Those factors, however, make them roughly equivalent in the long run. That's why there are roughly equal numbers of men and women in the world.

Sperm are really, really small. While it might not seem like a big deal to travel from the vagina to the egg, the truth of the matter is that it's a long journey. When a man ejaculates, he usually deposits about 250 million sperm into the vagina. Of those, though, it's thought that fewer than 100 actually make it all the way to the egg.

The fastest sperm might make it to the egg in thirty minutes. But it's also possible for fertilization to happen five days after sex. In the thirty-minute version, we imagine it's more likely a boy and in the five-day version, it's more likely a girl. The problem is, there's no way to select for one of these two occurrences. You can't make conception happen in thirty minutes any more than you can make it happen in five days. Certainly, the position in which sex occurs has no effect on this. After all, the differences in where ejaculation occurs in different positions are incredibly small compared to other factors. How quickly conception happens after sex is determined by many, many, many other factors, one of which is certainly luck.

This won't stop many of you from trying different positions in your efforts to influence the sex of your children. The problem is that about half of the time, you will "succeed." When that happens, you'll start telling your friends about it—and another myth will be born.

You Can't Get Pregnant If . . .

H ere's the thing about getting pregnant. If there's a sperm and an egg, and there's some way for the sperm to get to the egg, you can get pregnant. Period. There are all sorts of ways that people think they are safe from getting pregnant. They're almost all myths. Here are some of the most popular:

You can't get pregnant if he pulls out before he comes.

Close contact between a penis and a vagina can lead to pregnancy. Period. If a guy pulls his penis out before he comes, it still may be too late.

Before a man actually ejaculates or climaxes, there are usually drops of semen at the end of the penis. These drops of semen help to lubricate the head of the penis and may be present before a man feels close to coming. Even one drop of semen can contain a million sperm. And it only takes one sperm. It's completely possible for one of the sperm out of that drop of semen to make it to the egg. Furthermore, the seconds before climax are not the best time to expect someone to use good judgment and pull out. Studies show that when 100 women use this method to prevent pregnancy, 23 will end up getting pregnant within a year. In the very, very best scenario for using withdrawal, 16 in 100 get pregnant. These odds suck.

Other studies confirm that lots of people get pregnant using the withdrawal method. In a study of 1,910 women in Turkey (where 35 percent of the group was using coitus interruptus or pulling out to try to prevent pregnancy), 38 percent of the women had at least one unwanted pregnancy. In a study from a family planning association in Mauritius, where about 30 percent of the population is reported to use coitus interruptus as their method of choice, 34 percent of people indicated that they or their partner had become pregnant while relying on withdrawal.

Along these lines, you can also get pregnant if he doesn't put it all the way in. First of all, if he puts it partway in, but ejaculates, a woman would have lots and lots of sperm inside of her that can still try their luck at swimming up to an egg. Second, even if he didn't come inside, you still may have some small drops of semen with their millions of sperm, also swimming along and trying their luck at finding the egg. Even if the drops of semen are just close to the girl's vagina, there is a chance that a sperm will sneak inside and make its way to the egg. Again, it just takes one.

You can't get pregnant if you have sex while standing up.

Do people actually still believe this? You can get pregnant in any position. The egg and sperm can move and can join together no matter what position your body is in. Gravity doesn't make a big difference. It is possible that it might make it somewhat less likely for the sperm to find their way up to the egg in the fallopian tubes, but it is still very, very possible that they will.

Have you ever seen a sperm? This is why sperm have those crazy little tails that help them swim—so they can beat gravity or even the tide, so to speak. There are 300 million sperm in every 3 to 5 mL of ejaculate fluid, and they are all programmed with one mission in mind, to swim toward the uterus. Feel free to jump up and down or stand up all day; you may manage to deter a few of the sperm in their quest, but millions will still be swimming in search of the egg.

If over 20 percent of people are still getting pregnant when the penis is pulled out and most of the ejaculate is outside of the vagina, how much do you think standing up will decrease your odds?

You can't get pregnant if you have sex in the water.

You can get pregnant if you have unprotected sex, no matter where you do it. If a penis is in a vagina, then it really doesn't matter what's going on anywhere else. Warm water, cold water, chemically treated water—none of these will make a difference. You are just as likely to get pregnant during sex in the water as during sex out of the water. Granted, if a man ejaculates in the water, it is pretty unlikely that the sperm will find their way into the vagina and up to the egg, but it's not impossible, either. Plus, it's likely that some sperm will slip out no matter how hard a man tries not to let that happen (see pulling out above).

You can't get pregnant when you're on the pill.

Birth control pills work a lot better to prevent pregnancy than any of the other methods we have talked about. Much, much better than standing up. Much better than trying to pull out. Much better than restricting your activities to the hot tub. But the pill is not perfect, either. Again, if there is a sperm and an egg involved, pregnancy is always a possibility.

In the course of a year, 5 to 8 out of 100 women using the pill will have an accidental pregnancy. Those are better odds than for other methods (remember, it was 23 out of 100 women getting pregnant using the withdrawal method), but it's not down to 0. Birth control pills work best when a woman takes them every single day at the exact same time of day. If you take the pills absolutely perfectly, you are even less likely to get pregnant. But if you are not good at taking a pill every day and at the same time every day, your chance of getting pregnant while using the pill is higher. Missing even one day of the pill can significantly increase your chance of getting pregnant.

Part Five

SEXUALLY TRANSMITTED INFECTIONS

You Didn't Get That STD from Sex

A lot of people believe that they might get a sexually transmitted disease (STD) from a toilet seat. The fear of toilet
seats springs from the idea that public toilets are filthy places
full of bacteria. Plus, your private parts just might rub up
against something on that seat. It seems a lot easier to blame
the toilet than to blame your boyfriend.

When we refer to "sexually transmitted diseases," we are
talking about infections caused by either bacteria or viruses
that are typically passed only when one person has sex or
contact with the sexual organs of another person. These are
diseases like chlamydia, gonorrhea, herpes, and HIV. The
scary idea that you could get one of these serious infections
from a toilet seat is enough to make anyone want to hover
over the toilet bowl. It also offers a convenient excuse for how
you may have gotten one of these infections without sex being involved.

There is no research proving that people get infected with
sexually transmitted diseases from sitting on toilet seats. This
does not mean that it is impossible to get infected from a toilet seat, but there is no evidence either way. There are a few
published cases where physicians describe patients who they
believe may have become infected after direct contact with
exceptionally dirty toilet seats, but in these cases, they cannot
prove that the patients did not have physical or sexual contact of some kind with a person who was infected. The

majority of experts, including the president of the American Society for Microbiology, report never seeing or hearing about cases of people actually acquiring an STD from a toilet seat (unless they were having sex with another person while on the toilet!).

Even though it may be theoretically possible to get infected from a toilet seat, there are many reasons why this is very unlikely to actually happen. First of all, most of the bugs that cause sexually transmitted diseases in humans do not survive well outside of the human body. The viruses that cause herpes and AIDS do not live outside of the body for long. They dry out and die when exposed to air, and there have been no proven cases of people getting herpes or AIDS from a toilet seat. The bacteria that cause infections like chlamydia and gonorrhea do not live much longer.

Second, to get the bugs onto the toilet seat, someone would first need to leave their bodily fluids on the toilet seat. Obviously, public toilet seats do end up with a lot of urine on them, but urine is not where these germs live. These germs live in the fluids in your vagina or penis, or sometimes in your blood. It is much less likely that someone would be rubbing against a toilet seat or sitting in a way that would leave discharge or secretions from their vagina or penis on the seat. And usually, people do not ejaculate or bleed onto the toilet seat.

Moreover, even if the bug *did* get onto the seat in one of these secretions and did manage to survive, it is not a sure thing that someone coming into contact with that bug-infested fluid would become infected. In fact, it is quite unlikely. The bugs would have to be transferred from the seat into your urethra or to your genital tract, or maybe into a cut or sore somewhere on your private parts. You would need to touch the gunk on the toilet seat with one of these parts. Do you realize how unlikely it is that you would do that? Very unlikely.

Finally, even if someone did leave a germ, it survived, and you touched it, there very well might not be enough of the germs to cause you an infection. For many of these infections, you need to come in contact with a pretty large number of the bugs to make you sick. While it is theoretically possible that just one or two germs might infect you, it is incredibly unlikely.

But What About Crabs? I Know You Can Get Those from the Toilet Seat!

With any hope, you can see why it is awfully difficult to get a sexually transmitted bacteria or virus from the toilet seat, but you might be wondering about those little bugs that creep and crawl and jump. Could you get crabs or scabies from a toilet seat?

Crabs are lice that live in your pubic hair. They are a different type of lice than the lice that live in the hair on your head, but they cause lots of itching and irritation. Just like the lice that live in the hair on your head, pubic lice are very contagious. Crabs or pubic lice are probably the infection that you could get the most easily from a toilet seat. This has not been studied well, and it would be very, very rare, but it is possible that you could get crabs from a toilet seat. Pubic lice can live for about twenty-four hours when not on a human body, so they would not live there very long, but it is possible that one might wait on a toilet seat to infect you. Again, this is very unlikely, but the experts say it's possible.

Scabies is somewhat similar to crabs in that it is an itchy skin disease caused by little bugs called mites. Scabies can be spread through sexual contact or through being skin-to-skin or very close to someone with scabies. Experts also say that it might be possible to contract scabies if the mites are left on the toilet seat. This is, again, very unlikely, as things like close hugging or handshaking, are only very rarely a way that people get infected with scabies. Scabies can live off of the body longer than some other bugs, but they still only live for about twenty-four to thirty-six hours outside of the human body.

Toilet seats are pretty gross, but your risk of getting any sort of infection from a toilet seat is incredibly low. This risk is even lower for a sexually transmitted infection! You would be much, much better off using a condom regularly with your partners than worrying obsessively about the toilet seat. Not having sex is also a much more effective way to avoid sexually transmitted diseases than avoiding public toilets. While it might be reasonable to clean off the toilet seat with a wad of toilet paper or to try to squat without touching one, the most important advice is to wash your hands after using the bathroom and practice safe sex!

Oral Sex Is Totally Safe

Speaking of safe sex. . . . Safe sex is a very good thing. (We are certain Martha Stewart would agree.) Unfortunately, many people really do not know how to have safe sex. While a lot of people know that vaginal sex or anal sex can be dangerous, they think that oral sex is safer.

Oral sex is definitely safer in terms of pregnancy. Giving or receiving oral sex has no risk of getting you pregnant. Getting pregnant requires a sperm to come in contact with an egg inside of a woman. No one is going to get pregnant during oral sex unless you somehow get some semen in contact with the woman's vagina in the midst of oral sex (Aaron wants to hear how you think that will happen.)

While toilet seats are quite safe in terms of STDs, oral sex is not nearly as safe. You can get an STD from oral sex, whether you are on the giving end or the receiving end, and whether you are male or female. Infections like herpes, gonorrhea, and chlamydia can all spread that way. Both bacteria and viruses can spread from one person to another through oral sex. The virus that causes genital warts and cervical cancer, human papillomavirus, can even spread through oral sex. Do you remember how the actor Michael Douglas blamed his throat cancer on pleasuring his partners with oral sex? Yes, that's possible.

The person whose mouth is in contact with the genitals can get infections or sores in their own mouth from performing oral sex on someone with one of these infections. And if the person giving oral sex has an infection in their mouth, that infection can be passed to the person receiving the oral sex. This is especially common with oral herpes or cold sores. These infections can be passed even if your partner does not have any symptoms and you do not know that they are infected. (We know this sucks. No pun intended.)

The good news is that most of these infections do not spread as easily through oral sex as they do through vaginal or anal sex. You are much less likely to get herpes, gonorrhea, or chlamydia from oral sex than from these other forms of sex. While it is considered possible to get HIV from oral sex if the person has cuts or sores, experts say it is very unlikely that you would get HIV from oral sex, either. Nonetheless, it is possible. Even though it is a low risk, you can get HIV or gonorrhea or herpes from oral sex, especially if there is a cut or sore or something in the person's mouth.

Even if the risks from oral sex are not as high as the risks from other types of sex, the smartest thing is to protect yourself. First, talk with your partner about any infections either of you may have. For men, the penis could be covered with a latex condom. For women, the person giving oral sex could use some sort of protection to create a barrier between the mouth and the vagina. Examples of these kinds of barriers are called a dental dam or a latex sheet, or you could use a condom or even plastic wrap that is cut open to make a protective square. These same things can be used to create a barrier between the mouth and the anus for that kind of oral sex.

We know that the idea of having oral sex with these protective barriers in place does not sound like much fun.

However, the idea of getting throat infections, sores in your mouth, or even throat cancers sounds like much less fun. Even worse is the possibility that you could be infected with something like HIV. Play safely!

Condoms Will Protect You
from Anything

We love condoms. There is no doubt that, if you use a condom, you will decrease your chance of getting a sexually transmitted disease. Almost all of Rachel's work involves treating families with HIV, and she is constantly promoting condoms for just this reason. Condoms are an excellent way to protect yourself or your partner from HIV.

However, many people think condoms are 100 percent effective—in essence, many believe that you simply cannot get a sexually transmitted disease while wearing a condom. Unfortunately, that's just not true.

Now, this should never be a reason not to use a condom. They are *very* effective in preventing the transmission of certain diseases. For instance, a review of studies done on condom use to prevent gonorrhea found that using condoms reduced the risk of getting gonorrhea somewhere between 30 and 100 percent for males and between 13 and 100 percent for females. This is great! Similar studies looking at protection against chlamydia found that condom use reduced the risk of getting chlamydia somewhere between 15 and 100 percent for males and 10 and 100 percent for females. Again, hooray for condoms! (If you want to be on the higher side of those percentages—meaning you want the condom to reduce the risk of those infections by 100 percent—then you need to use the condom correctly every single time you have sex. If you use them properly, they work. . . .) Perhaps the most concerning sexually transmitted disease is the most studied—HIV. There is no doubt that using condoms will reduce your chance of getting of HIV, the virus that causes AIDS. Once again, very good news, and a very, very good reason to wear a condom.

A 2005 study examined how well condoms could prevent passing on the herpes simplex virus (HSV) to someone else. Of the 1,843 participants in the study, just over 6 percent became infected. Those using condoms were less likely to become infected with HSV-2 (one of the types of herpes), but condoms provided no protection against becoming infected with another type of herpes (HSV-1). And, if the herpes is in a spot that is not covered by a condom, the condom helps you even less.

There are even more sexually transmitted diseases that might affect areas not covered by condoms, things like human papillomavirus (which causes genital warts and cervical cancer), crabs (which scurry all around), and others like genital ulcers. If any of these things are not covered and protected by the condom, then they can be passed on to other people. Condoms are great, but again, they aren't perfect.

Part of this is due to human nature and plain old bad luck. In the lab, condoms were pretty much 100 percent effective in blocking the nasty bugs that cause sexually transmitted diseases. However, real life is not the same as what we see in the lab. As we said, the condoms don't cover up everything. Moreover, condoms can break, and if they do, you can pass on a disease (or knock someone up). And, of course, you need to use a condom every single time you have sex in order for them to be fully effective. We have yet to meet the mythical person who never, ever fails to use a condom.

None of this should be taken as a reason not to use condoms. They are still awesome at preventing the transmission of many sexually transmitted diseases, and using condoms is probably the safest way for you to have sex. You just have to realize that the condom is not perfect. You need to be smart about who you have sex with and what is on their genitals. You need to use a condom correctly for it to help you fully. And, if you have something that is not covered by a condom, you're not protected.

You Don't Need the HPV Vaccine If You're Not Having Sex

Human papillomavirus is a very common sexually transmitted infection, and lots of research links this virus to causing certain types of cancer. Getting the vaccine is the best way to prevent infection, and therefore the best way to prevent cancer. In order to prevent infection, though, the vaccine schedule needs to be completed before sex occurs for the first time.

The next obvious question is: How early is that? A lot of parents think their children are too young to need the HPV vaccine.

All parents (including Aaron) hope that their children will be responsible and not engage in sexual activity before they are ready. Pretending that none will, though, is somewhat ignorant. It ignores what most of us remember from our youth. More importantly, it ignores the available data and evidence.

Data show that children are having sex. Let's start with intercourse. There have been a number of studies that have examined at what age children have engaged in full-on sex. A study from the Guttmacher Institute in 2002 found that, by the end of their teenage years, more than three-quarters of all adolescents—both boys and girls—had engaged in sexual intercourse. More than two-thirds of them had had sex with at least two people.

The average age of first intercourse in this study was less

than seventeen years for boys and less than seventeen-and-a-half years for girls.

A more detailed study was published in 2005 by the CDC. This one broke things down more by age. By fifteen years of age, about a quarter of both boys and girls had engaged in sexual intercourse. Given the prevalence and the infectivity of HPV, this means that a lot of children younger than fifteen would be infected with HPV unless they had finished the full course of vaccines long before then.

A more recent report from the CDC, from their 2011 Youth Risk Behavior Surveillance System survey, found that more than 6 percent of children in the United States had sexual intercourse before the age of thirteen. This included 9 percent of males and more than 3 percent of females. We are sure that most parents think this number is much too high, and that most parents cannot imagine their own children having sex this young. But that doesn't change the facts. Children have sex, and often those who are "too young" are the ones most likely to forgo protection. In fact, about two in five sexually active children report that they did not use a condom the last time they had sex. They're not adequately protecting themselves.

If children this young are having sex, then we need to vaccinate them even younger. There are almost 19 million newly diagnosed sexually transmitted infections each year, and more than half of them occur in teens and young adults age fifteen to twenty-four years old.

Vaginal intercourse also isn't the only type of sex that kids engage in. On top of the numbers above, another 7 percent of girls and 9 percent of boys have performed or received oral sex even though they haven't tried vaginal intercourse. HPV can be passed along through any kind of sex—oral, vaginal, or anal.

The bottom line is that the vaccine is preventive. It does no good once you've already got HPV. Children engage in sexual behaviors at young ages, and the point of a vaccine program is to protect all of them. To do so, we need to start giving the vaccine at an age that is surprising to some, but necessary to get in front of all of this. In the long run, we're trying to prevent cancer. If we could remove the sexual aspects from this, it would likely be easier for many parents to swallow. Giving the vaccine does not imply consent for children to have sex. It just protects children.

The HPV Vaccine Encourages Girls to Have Sex

Vaccines can be surprisingly controversial. Any of them that touch on sexual activity at all are even more so. This holds true for the vaccine for the human papillomavirus. Since 2006, the CDC has recommended that all girls in the United States who are ages eleven to twelve receive the immunization. It can be administered to girls as young as nine years.

Why? Human papillomavirus is the leading cause of cervical cancer. This is a cancer that kills 4,000 women each year in the United States. And it causes many, many thousands more deaths worldwide. About 15,000 HPV-associated cancers could be prevented each year if we vaccinated everyone. HPV is a very common sexually transmitted infection that causes genital warts.

The reason that the vaccine is recommended for girls age eleven and twelve is that the vaccine only works if you need to have all three doses before you might be exposed to HPV. Therefore, we want to get girls through the complete series well before they have sex. You can catch HPV even the first time you have sex, so you want to get out in front of this in terms of vaccination.

This vaccine is known to be very safe. By mid-2012, it had been given more than 46 million times in the United States. No significant adverse effects have been noted. While there isn't even any evidence that the vaccine is dangerous for pregnant women, to be on the safe side, pregnant women don't routinely receive it.

Even with all of this, some people still oppose the widespread administration of this vaccine to young girls. Some believe that giving a vaccine that prevents a sexually transmitted infection implicitly encourages girls to have sex. They feel like giving the vaccine is a moral issue that is best decided on an individual basis. The problem is that, in general, parents don't have much control over the sexual activities of their children. At least, they don't have so much control that it's worth taking a chance with this infection.

But forget all of this. The concern that giving the vaccine makes girls more likely to have sex is a testable hypothesis. In fact, a study on exactly this point has been conducted. In 2012, researchers published a manuscript that reported on a cohort of almost 1,400 girls, 493 who had received the vaccine. They followed them for three years after immunization to see if there were any differences in sexual outcomes.

There weren't any. The girls who got the vaccine didn't get any more sexually transmitted infections, didn't get pregnant more often, and didn't seek contraceptive counseling more.

But we're not doing that great a job. By 2011, only about a third of girls age thirteen to seventeen years were immunized against HPV. That was barely more than the 32 percent who were vaccinated in 2010. We must do better. Think of it this way—we have a vaccine that can actually prevent a certain kind of cancer! Let's take advantage of that incredible opportunity and make sure that we protect girls and women.

It's also important to remember that the HPV vaccine is

recommended for boys as well. HPV can cause more than cervical cancer. It can cause other cancers, many of which are more prevalent in male populations, as well as genital warts. It's going to become more important than ever that we overcome myths about this vaccine in order to do the most good.

You Better Not Kiss
Anyone with HIV

When she is not writing books about medical myths, Rachel spends all of her time working on research related to HIV or taking care of children who are infected with HIV. Because of this focus, Rachel cares very, very much about debunking myths related to HIV.

HIV remains one of the world's most serious health challenges. Around the world, 34 million people are living with HIV right now, including 3.4 million children. In the countries that make up sub-Saharan Africa, almost 1 in 20 adults is infected with HIV. And far, far too many people are still dying from HIV—1.7 million deaths in 2011 alone.

It makes sense to be worried about getting infected with HIV; it is a serious infection for which we do not yet have a vaccine or a cure. We do have very good medicines that can keep the HIV virus under control so that HIV-infected people can live long, healthy, and productive lives, but preventing new infections is still a much better plan. Worldwide, we are actually doing a pretty good job of stopping HIV from being passed from one person to another. Between 2001 and 2011, the number of new HIV infections each year decreased by 20 percent.

How does someone get infected with HIV? HIV lives in blood and other body fluids, including saliva, semen, and vaginal fluid. By far, the most common way that HIV is passed from one person to another is through sexual activity, including both vaginal intercourse and anal intercourse. HIV is also passed from mothers to babies during pregnancy, at the time of delivery, and through breast milk.

We can almost completely stop HIV infections through a few easy steps. Using condoms protects you from getting HIV during vaginal or anal intercourse. If the HIV-infected person is taking medicines for HIV and has suppressed the amount of virus in their blood, then this also makes it very unlikely that you will be infected from them. If pregnant women and mothers who are breast-feeding take the medicines that fight HIV, then less than 1 percent of their babies will be infected. We can actually stop almost all of these infections. Imagine if we could stop 1.7 million a people a year from dying. Imagine having a generation of babies that are HIV-free. What a wonderful thing!

We usually counsel people that you cannot get HIV from casual contact with an infected person. Kissing, hugging, shaking hands, sharing food, drinking from the same cup—most doctors (Rachel included) will tell you that these activities are not going to pass HIV from one person to another.

It is very, very unlikely that any of the activities on that list—including kissing—would allow you to get HIV. But what about oral sex? Or any other kinds of kissing? HIV does live in the saliva, and so we have to wonder about whether you can get HIV from someone's mouth. One also should wonder whether you could get an HIV infection into your own mouth. Just because a virus lives in saliva does not mean that it can infect you from saliva, so knowing that HIV is in saliva does not answer the question alone.

A 2006 review examined the question of "oral transmission,"

looking at studies on whether HIV can pass through oral sex (in either direction) or through other activities involving the mouth. The combined studies suggest that it is very, very unlikely that HIV would pass to another person through saliva alone or mouth-to-mouth contact. Multiple studies show no transmission through kissing or sharing utensils or dishes.

Oral sex, however, can transmit HIV. It's rare for HIV to be passed between people this way (much less common than through genital-to-genital sex or genital-to-anus sex), but it's possible. There have been reports of a handful of cases in which HIV was transmitted to people who performed oral sex on an infected partner. The highest risk in oral sex is for the person performing the fellatio, meaning the person with their mouth on the genitals or anus (the technical term is "active oral-genital contact"). There is a risk, albeit small, that this person would contract HIV in through their mouth from the person on whom they are performing oral sex. This risk goes up if the person has sores or cuts of any sort inside of their mouth. We wish we could say that there is no HIV risk from oral sex, but there is a small one.

Even though it is *possible* for HIV to be passed in this way, this is still a very, very uncommon event. Large studies have followed couples where one partner was infected and the other was not infected to see whether and how HIV transmissions occurred. In one of these ten-year studies, despite 263 couples having unprotected oral sex over 19,000 times during this time period (10,295 giving oral sex and 10,658 receiving oral sex), there were no cases in which HIV was passed from the infected partner to the other person. None. And these are couples where we know one of the partners was infected the entire time.

The oral cavity has a number of features that make it resistant to HIV. The cells that line the walls of the oral cavity are thick and resistant to HIV infections. The immune cells that HIV targets for infection (CD4 cells) are relatively scarce in the mouth. And the saliva actually contains a lot of antibodies against viruses, as well as other chemicals that are protective against HIV. Fourteen different components of the saliva have been reported to have a protective activity against HIV.

While all of these things keep the mouth very safe overall, even the body's best defenses are not always enough when a very large amount of HIV is present (as might happen if someone who is not on HIV treatment ejaculates in your mouth) or when something like a cold sore or cut in the mouth gives the virus a weak spot through which to sneak into the bloodstream.

The summary is that oral sex is much, much less risky for getting HIV than other kinds of sex, but there is still a small risk of getting HIV this way.

Anal Sex Will Give You Cancer

Let's address another concern about anal sex. It's the idea that anal sex will give you cancer. Unfortunately, as with a number of myths, there's a kernel of truth in here, and that's just powerful enough to give this idea legs. But it's worth unpacking the nuances of why anal sex is *associated* with cancer, and why you should know about it.

We're not going to repeat everything we said about anal sex before. But given the fact that many people still think of it as "dirty" or "taboo" for a variety of reasons, there are some negative stereotypes associated with the act that persist even in light of evidence.

The biggest truth here is that the incidence of anal and rectal cancer is increasing. A 2010 study looking at the Surveillance, Epidemiology, and End Results (SEER) cancer registry, which carefully tracks the incidence of cancers, showed that rectal cancer has been going up by 2 to 3 percent per year for decades in people less than forty years of age. There have been no similar increases in colon cancer.

While the authors of this study noting this increase in rectal cancers did not suggest that anal sex was to blame, many others jumped to that conclusion. Many immediately blamed the increased acceptance of anal intercourse for this finding. In fact, there was a letter to the editor about the initial study explicitly making this link. The authors responded, correctly, that there are no data in SEER to back up this claim, and that while it's certainly worthy of study, it is a leap too far to blame anal sex for this finding.

But there's little doubt that anal sex is associated with anal or rectal cancer. That's a subtle difference, but it's critical.

Having anal sex makes it more likely to spread sexually transmitted infections, like the human papillomavirus. Infection with this virus is believed to lead to a number of cancers. When you have anal sex, especially when unprotected, then you are more likely to cause small anal fissures, which can increase the risk of HPV infection.

This same argument holds, of course, for HPV transmission to women through vaginal intercourse, and the subsequent risk of cervical cancer (also caused by HPV). This link is well understood and accepted. There is even a vaccine now for HPV to prevent the subsequent cervical cancer that can follow infection with HPV. It was initially intended for girls (to prevent cervical cancer). Now recommendations are extending to boys, to prevent rectal or anal cancer.

But does anyone say that vaginal intercourse *causes* cervical cancer? Of course not. We blame the virus, not the act.

If people without STDs engage in safe sex, even anal sex, there really is no increased risk of anal or rectal cancer. At least, there's no risk documented in any studies we could find. The risks are the same for all STDs and cancers associated with them. People who practice unsafe sex, especially with multiple partners, are at risk. It doesn't matter where you're putting things, or with whom. It's not anal sex that is your real problem. It's unsafe sex that's the risk.

Until we start blaming heterosexual vaginal intercourse for causing cancers related to STDs, it seems somewhat judgmental and unfair to blame anal sex for the same mechanisms of disease.

The bottom line is that all sex carries with it some risk of STD transmission, even if it is small. Anal sex causes cancer no more than vaginal sex does. In both, safety and thoughtfulness are your best protection against cancer.

References

PART I: MEN

Penis Size Matters

Bondil, P., P. Costa, J. P. Daures, J. F. Louis, and H. Navratil. "Clinical Study of the Longitudinal Deformation of the Flaccid Penis and of Its Variations with Aging." *European Urology* 21, no. 4 (1992): 284–86.

Costa, Rui Miguel, Geoffrey F. Miller, and Stuart Brody. "Women Who Prefer Longer Penises Are More Likely to Have Vaginal Orgasms (but Not Clitoral Orgasms): Implications for an Evolutionary Theory of Vaginal Orgasm." *Journal of Sexual Medicine* 9, no. 12 (2012): 3079–88.

Grov, Christian, Jeffrey T. Parsons, and David S. Bimbi. "The Association between Penis Size and Sexual Health among Men Who Have Sex with Men." *Archives of Sexual Behavior* 39, no. 3 (2010): 788–97.

Jamison, Paul L., and Paul H. Gebhard. "Penis Size Increase between Flaccid and Erect States: An Analysis of the Kinsey Data." *The Journal of Sex Research* 24 (1988): 177–83.

Lever, Janet, David A. Frederick, and Letitia Anne Peplau. "Does Size Matter? Men's and Women's Views on Penis Size across the Lifespan." *Psychology of Men & Masculinity* 7, no. 3 (2006): 129–43.

Mautz, Brian S., Bob B. M. Wong, Richard A. Peters, and Michael D. Jennions. "Penis Size Interacts with Body Shape and Height to Influence Male Attractiveness." *Proceedings of the National Academy of Sciences* 110, no. 17 (2013): 6925–30.

Pierce, Aaron Paul. "The Coital Alignment Technique (Cat): An Overview of Studies." *Journal of Sex & Marital Therapy* 26, no. 3 (2000): 257–68.

Schonfeld, W. A., Beebe, G. W. "Normal Growth and Variation in the Male Genitalia from Birth to Maturity." *Journal of Urology* 48 (1942): 759.

Wessells, H., T. F. Lue, and J. W. McAninch. "Penile Length in the Flaccid and Erect States: Guidelines for Penile Augmentation." *Journal of Urology* 156, no. 3 (1996): 995–97.

Wikipedia. "Coital Alignment Technique." http://en.wikipedia.org/wiki/Coital _alignment_technique.

Batters Up! The Battle of the 7-Inch Penis.

Awwad, Z., M. Abu-Hijleh, S. Basri, N. Shegam, M. Murshidi, and K. Ajlouni. "Penile Measurements in Normal Adult Jordanians and in Patients with Erectile Dysfunction." *International Journal of Impotence Research* 17, no. 2 (2005): 191–95.

Bondil, P., P. Costa, J. P. Daures, J. F. Louis, and H. Navratil. "Clinical Study of the Longitudinal Deformation of the Flaccid Penis and of Its Variations with Aging." *Europenan Urology* 21, no. 4 (1992): 284–86.

Chen, J., A. Gefen, A. Greenstein, H. Matzkin, and D. Elad. "Predicting Penile Size During Erection." *International Journal of Impotence Research* 12, no. 6 (2000): 328–33.

Edwards, R. "The Definitive Penis Size Survey." http://www.sizesurvey.com/quest.html.

Herbenick, D., M. Reece, V. Schick, and S. Sanders. "Erect Penile Length and Circumference Dimensions of 1,661 Sexually Active Men in the United States." *Journal of Sexual Medicine* (2013). doi: 10.1111/jsm.12244.

Khan, Shahid, Bhaskar Somani, Wayne Lam, and Roland Donat. "Establishing a Reference Range for Penile Length in Caucasian British Men: A Prospective Study of 609 Men." *BJU International* 109, no. 5 (2012): 740–44.

Mehraban, D., M. Salehi, and F. Zayeri. "Penile Size and Somatometric Parameters among Iranian Normal Adult Men." *International Journal of Impotence Research* 19, no. 3 (2007): 303–9.

Mondaini, N., R. Ponchietti, P. Gontero, G. H. Muir, A. Natali, F. Di Loro, E. Caldarera, S. Biscioni, and M. Rizzo. "Penile Length Is Normal in Most Men Seeking Penile Lengthening Procedures." *International Journal of Impotence Research* 14, no. 4 (2002): 283.

Ponchietti, R., N. Mondaini, M. Bonafe, F. Di Loro, S. Biscioni, and L. Masieri. "Penile Length and Circumference: A Study on 3,300 Young Italian Males." *European Urology* 39, no. 2 (2001): 183–86.

Promodu, K., K. V. Shanmughadas, S. Bhat, and K. R. Nair. "Penile Length and Circumference: An Indian Study." *International Journal of Impotence Research* 19, no. 6 (2007): 558–63.

Schneider, T., H. Sperling, G. Lümmen, J. Syllwasschy, and H. Rübben. "Does Penile Size in Younger Men Cause Problems in Condom Use? A Prospective Measurement of Penile Dimensions in 111 Young and 32 Older Men." *Urology* 57, no. 2 (2001): 314–18.

Schonfeld, W. A., Beebe, G. W., "Normal Growth and Variation in the Male Genitalia from Birth to Maturity." *Journal of Urology* 48 (1942): 759.

Sengezer, Mustafa, Serdar Oztürk, and Mustafa Deveci. "Accurate Method for Determining Functional Penile Length in Turkish Young Men." *Annals of Plastic Surgery* 48, no. 4 (2002): 381–85.

Shamloul, Rany. "Treatment of Men Complaining of Short Penis." *Urology* 65, no. 6 (2005): 1183–85.

Son, H., H. Lee, J. S. Huh, S. W. Kim, and J. S. Paick. "Studies on Self-Esteem of Penile Size in Young Korean Military Men." *Asian Journal of Andrology* 5, no. 3 (2003): 185–89.

Spyropoulos, Evangelos, Dimitrios Borousas, Stamatios Mavrikos, Athanasios Dellis, Michael Bourounis, and Sotirios Athanasiadis. "Size of External

Genital Organs and Somatometric Parameters among Physically Normal Men Younger Than 40 Years Old." *Urology* 60, no. 3 (2002): 485–89.

Wessells, H., T. F. Lue, and J. W. McAninch. "Penile Length in the Flaccid and Erect States: Guidelines for Penile Augmentation." *Journal of Urology* 156, no. 3 (1996): 995–97.

Big Feet, Big Hands, Big . . . ?

Cobb, John, and Denis Duboule. "Comparative Analysis of Genes Downstream of the Hoxd Cluster in Developing Digits and External Genitalia." *Development (Cambridge, England)* 132, no. 13 (2005): 3055–67.

Edwards, R. "The Definitive Penis Size Survey." http://www.sizesurvey.com/quest.html.

Shah, J., and N. Christopher. "Can Shoe Size Predict Penile Length?" *BJU International* 90, no. 6 (2002): 586–87.

Siminoski, Kerry, and Jerald Bain. "The Relationships among Height, Penile Length, and Foot Size." *Sexual Abuse: A Journal of Research and Treatment* 6, no. 3 (1993): 231–35.

Racial Penis Profiling

Lynn, Richard. "Rushton's R-K Life History Theory of Race Differences in Penis Length and Circumference Examined in 113 Populations." *Personality and Individual Differences* 55, no. 3 (2013): 261–66.

Rushton, J. Philippe. *Race, Evolution and Behavior.* New Brunswick, NJ: Transaction Publishers, 1995, 9–46.

You Don't Last Long Enough

Althof, S. E., C. H. Abdo, J. Dean, G. Hackett, M. McCabe, C. G. McMahon, R. C. Rosen, R. Sadovsky, M. Waldinger, E. Becher, G. A. Broderick, J. Buvat, I. Goldstein, A. I. El-Meliegy, F. Giuliano, W. J. Hellstrom, L. Incrocci, E. A. Jannini, K. Park, S. Parish, H. Porst, D. Rowland, R. Segraves, I. Sharlip, C. Simonelli, and H. M. Tan. "International Society for Sexual Medicine's Guidelines for the Diagnosis and Treatment of Premature Ejaculation." *Journal of Sexual Medicine* 7, no. 9 (2010): 2947–69.

Kinsey, Alfred C., Wardell B. Pomeroy, and Clyde E. Martin. "Sexual Behavior in the Human Male." *Journal of Nervous and Mental Disease* 109, no. 3 (1949): 283.

McMahon, Chris G., Carmita Abdo, Luca Incrocci, Michael Perelman, David Rowland, Marcel Waldinger, and Zhong Cheng Xin. "Disorders of Orgasm and Ejaculation in Men." *Journal of Sexual Medicine* 1, no. 1 (2004): 58–65.

Mulhall, J. P. "Premature Ejaculation." *Campbell-Walsh Urology.* Philadelphia, PA: Saunders Elsevier, 2011.

Waldinger, M. D., P. Quinn, M. Dilleen, R. Mundayat, D. H. Schweitzer, and

M. Boolell. "A Multinational Population Survey of Intravaginal Ejaculation Latency Time." *Journal of Sexual Medicine* 2, no. 4 (2005): 492–97.

You Shouldn't Have Sex Before the Big Game

McGlone, S., and I. Shrier. "Does Sex the Night before Competition Decrease Performance?" *Clinical Journal of Sport Medicine* 10, no. 4 (2000): 233–34.

Foreskin and Seven Years Ago . . .

Bronselaer, G. A., J. M. Schober, H. F. Meyer-Bahlburg, G. T'Sjoen, R. Vlietinck, and P. B. Hoebeke. "Male Circumcision Decreases Penile Sensitivity as Measured in a Large Cohort." *BJU International* 111, no. 5 (2013): 820–27.

Gray, R. H., G. Kigozi, D. Serwadda, F. Makumbi, F. Nalugoda, S. Watya, L. Moulton, M. Z. Chen, N. K. Sewankambo, N. Kiwanuka, V. Sempijja, T. Lutalo, J. Kagayii, F. Wabwire-Mangen, R. Ridzon, M. Bacon, and M. J. Wawer. "The Effects of Male Circumcision on Female Partners' Genital Tract Symptoms and Vaginal Infections in a Randomized Trial in Rakai, Uganda." *American Journal of Obstetrics & Gynecology* 200, no. 1 (2009): 42.e1–7.

Kigozi, G., S. Watya, C. B. Polis, D. Buwembo, V. Kiggundu, M. J. Wawer, D. Serwadda, F. Nalugoda, N. Kiwanuka, M. C. Bacon, V. Ssempijja, F. Makumbi, and R. H. Gray. "The Effect of Male Circumcision on Sexual Satisfaction and Function, Results from a Randomized Trial of Male Circumcision for Human Immunodeficiency Virus Prevention, Rakai, Uganda." *BJU International* 101, no. 1 (2008): 65–70.

Krieger, J. N., S. D. Mehta, R. C. Bailey, K. Agot, J. O. Ndinya-Achola, C. Parker, and S. Moses. "Adult Male Circumcision: Effects on Sexual Function and Sexual Satisfaction in Kisumu, Kenya." *Journal of Sexual Medicine* 5, no. 11 (2008): 2610–22.

Liu, C. M., B. A. Hungate, A. A. Tobian, D. Serwadda, J. Ravel, R. Lester, G. Kigozi, M. Aziz, R. M. Galiwango, F. Nalugoda, T. L. Contente-Cuomo, M. J. Wawer, P. Keim, R. H. Gray, and L. B. Price. "Male Circumcision Significantly Reduces Prevalence and Load of Genital Anaerobic Bacteria." *mBio* 4, no. 2 (2013): e00076.

Morris, B. J., J. N. Krieger, and G. Kigozi. "Male Circumcision Decreases Penile Sensitivity as Measured in a Large Cohort." *BJU International* 111, no. 5 (2013): E269–70.

Payne, K., L. Thaler, T. Kukkonen, S. Carrier, and Y. Binik. "Sensation and Sexual Arousal in Circumcised and Uncircumcised Men." *Journal of Sexual Medicine* 4, no. 3 (2007): 667–74.

Tian, Y., W. Liu, J. Z. Wang, R. Wazir, X. Yue, and K. J. Wang. "Effects of Circumcision on Male Sexual Functions: A Systematic Review and Meta-Analysis." *Asian Journal of Andrology* 15, no. 5 (2013): 662–66.

UNAIDS/WHO. "Male Circumcision: Global Trends and Determinants of Prevalence, Safety, and Acceptability." 2007.

Your Balls Sag with Age

Harris, I. D., C. Fronczak, L. Roth, and R. B. Meacham. "Fertility and the Aging Male." *Reviews in Urology* 13, no. 4 (2011): e184–90.

Hermann, M., G. Untergasser, H. Rumpold, and P. Berger. "Aging of the Male Reproductive System." *Experimental Gerontology* 35, no. 9–10 (2000): 1267–79.

WebMD. "Teen Boys." http://teens.webmd.com/boys/testicles-faq.

Wait for a Whopping Wad

Pound, N., M. H. Javed, C. Ruberto, M. A. Shaikh, and A. P. Del Valle. "Duration of Sexual Arousal Predicts Semen Parameters for Masturbatory Ejaculates." *Physiology & Behavior* 76, no. 4–5 (2002): 685–89.

Rehan, N., A. J. Sobrero, and J. W. Fertig. "The Semen of Fertile Men: Statistical Analysis of 1300 Men." *Fertility and Sterility* 26, no. 6 (1975): 492–502.

Start Small, Stay Small

Jamison, Paul L., and Paul H. Gebhard. "Penis Size Increase between Flaccid and Erect States: An Analysis of the Kinsey Data." *Journal of Sex Research* 24 (1988): 177–83.

Masters W. H., and V. E Johnson. *Human Sexual Response.* Boston: Little, Brown, 1966.

Wessells, Hunter, Tom F. Lue, and Jack W. McAninch. "Penile Length in the Flaccid and Erect States: Guidelines for Penile Augmentation." *Journal of Urology* 156, no. 3 (1996): 995–97.

Don't Swallow Your Cum!

Duncan, M. W., and H. S. Thompson. "Proteomics of semen and its constituents." *Proteomics Clinical Applications* 1, no. 8 (2007): 861–75. doi: 10.1002/prca.200700228.

There's Always Semen When You're Screamin'

Koeman M., M. F. van Driel, W. C. Schultz, and H. J. Mensink. "Orgasm after Radical Prostatectomy." *British Journal of Urology* 77, no. 6 (1996): 861–64.

Shimizu F., M. Taguri, Y. Harada, Y. Matsuyama, K. Sase, and M. Fujime. "Impact of Dry Ejaculation Caused by Highly Selective Alpha1a-Blocker: Randomized, Double-Blind, Placebo-Controlled Crossover Pilot Study in Healthy Volunteer Men." *Journal of Sexual Medicine* 7, no. 3 (2010): 1277–83.

Woodhouse, C. R., J. M. Reilly, and G. Bahadur. "Sexual Function and Fertility in Patients Treated for Posterior Urethral Valves." *Journal of Urology* (1989): 586–88.

You're Going to Break That Boner!

Amit, A., K. Arun, B. Bharat, R. Navin, T. Sameer, and D. U. Shankar. "Penile Fracture and Associated Urethral Injury: Experience at a Tertiary Care Hospital." *Canadian Urological Association Journal* 7, no. 3–4 (2013): E168–70.

Garcia Gomez, B., J. Romero, F. Villacampa, A. Tejido, and R. Diaz. "Early Treatment of Penile Fractures: Our Experience." *Archivos Españoles de Urologia* 65, no. 7 (2012): 684–88.

Shetty, K., and I. Apakama. "Penile Fracture: Well Heard; Rarely Seen." *ANZ Journal of Surgery* 81, no. 12 (2011): 943–44.

You Are Going to Pump That Geyser Dry

Amann, R. P. "Considerations in Evaluating Human Spermatogenesis on the Basis of Total Sperm Per Ejaculate." *Journal of Andrology* 30, no. 6 (2009): 626–41.

———. "The Cycle of the Seminiferous Epithelium in Humans: A Need to Revisit?" *Journal of Andrology* 29, no. 5 (2008): 469–87.

Pound, N., M. H. Javed, C. Ruberto, M. A. Shaikh, and A. P. Del Valle. "Duration of Sexual Arousal Predicts Semen Parameters for Masturbatory Ejaculates." *Physiology & Behavior* 76, no. 4–5 (2002): 685–89.

PART II: WOMEN

Wearing a Bra Will Keep Your Boobs from Sagging

Ashizawa, K., A. Sugane, and T. Gunji. "Breast Form Changes Resulting from a Certain Brassiere." *Journal of Human Ergology (Tokyo)* 19, no. 1 (1990): 53–62.

MacGuill, D. "Women Better Off without Bras: French Study." http://www.thelocal.fr/page/view/breasts-better-off-without-bras-french-study#.UWgFJxlgPhV.

Mason, B. R., K. A. Page, and K. Fallon. "An Analysis of Movement and Discomfort of the Female Breast During Exercise and the Effects of Breast Support in Three Cases." *Journal of Science and Medicine in Sport* 2, no. 2 (1999): 134–44.

McGhee, D. E., and J. R. Steele. "Breast Elevation and Compression Decrease Exercise-Induced Breast Discomfort." *Medicine & Science in Sports & Exercise* 42, no. 7 (2010): 1333–38.

Morris, Harvey. "France Debates the Merits of the Bra." http://rendezvous.blogs.nytimes.com/2013/04/11/france-debates-the-merits-of-the-bra/.

Page, K. A., and J. R. Steele. "Breast Motion and Sports Brassiere Design. Implications for Future Research." *Sports Medicine* 27, no. 4 (1999): 205–11.

Women Don't Really Want Sex

ABC News. "The American Sex Survey: A Peek beneath the Sheets." 10/21/04.

Abdo, Carmita H. N., Ana L. R. Valadares, Waldemar M. Oliveira Jr., Marco T. Scanavino, and João Afif-Abdo. "Hypoactive Sexual Desire Disorder in a Population-Based Study of Brazilian Women: Associated Factors Classified According to Their Importance." *Menopause (New York, N.Y.)* 17, no. 6 (2010): 1114–21.

Bergner, D. *What Do Women Want?: Adventures in the Science of Family Desire.* New York: Ecco, 2013, 9–42, 109–64.

Brotto, Lori A., Johannes Bitzer, Ellen Laan, Sandra Leiblum, and Mijal Luria. "Women's Sexual Desire and Arousal Disorders." *Journal of Sexual Medicine* 7, no. 1 Pt. 2 (2010): 586–614.

Carvalho, Joana, and Pedro Nobre. "Predictors of Women's Sexual Desire: The Role of Psychopathology, Cognitive-Emotional Determinants, Relationship Dimensions, and Medical Factors." *Journal of Sexual Medicine* 7, no. 2 Pt. 2 (2010): 928–37.

Chivers, Meredith L., Michael C. Seto, Martin L. Lalumière, Ellen Laan, and Teresa Grimbos. "Agreement of Self-Reported and Genital Measures of Sexual Arousal in Men and Women: A Meta-Analysis." *Archives of Sexual Behavior* 39, no. 1 (2010): 5–56.

Chivers, Meredith L., and A. D. Timmers. "Effects of Gender and Relationship Context in Audio Narratives on Genital and Subjective Sexual Response in Heterosexual Women and Men." *Archives of Sexual Behavior* 41, no. 1 (2012): 185–97.

Laumann, E. O., A. Nicolosi, D. B. Glasser, A. Paik, C. Gingell, E. Moreira, and T. Wang. "Sexual Problems among Women and Men Aged 40–80 Y: Prevalence and Correlates Identified in the Global Study of Sexual Attitudes and Behaviors." *International Journal of Impotence Research* 17, no. 1 (2005): 39–57.

Suschinsky, Kelly D., Martin L. Lalumière, and Meredith L. Chivers. "Sex Differences in Patterns of Genital Sexual Arousal: Measurement Artifacts or True Phenomena?" *Archives of Sexual Behavior* 38, no. 4 (2009): 559–73.

Wallen, K., and E. A. Lloyd. "Female Sexual Arousal: Genital Anatomy and Orgasm in Intercourse." *Hormones and Behavior* 59, no. 5 (2011): 780–92.

Wallen, K., and Heather A. Rupp. "Women's Interest in Visual Sexual Stimuli Varies with Menstrual Cycle Phase at First Exposure and Predicts Later Interest." *Hormones and Behavior* 57, no. 2 (2010): 263–68.

Witting, Katarina, Pekka Santtila, Markus Varjonen, Patrick Jern, Ada Johansson, Bettina von der Pahlen, and Kenneth Sandnabba. "Female Sexual Dysfunction, Sexual Distress, and Compatibility with Partner." *Journal of Sexual Medicine* 5, no. 11 (2008): 2587–99.

Bald Is Best (The Bush Versus the Brazilian)

Armstrong, N. R., and J. D. Wilson. "Did the 'Brazilian' Kill the Pubic Louse?" *Sexually Transmitted Infections* 82, no. 3 (2006): 265–66.

DeMaria, A. L., and A. B. Berenson. "Prevalence and Correlates of Pubic Hair Grooming among Low-Income Hispanic, Black, and White Women." *Body Image* 10, no. 2 (2013): 226–31.

Dendle, Claire, Sheila Mulvey, Felicity Pyrlis, M. Lindsay Grayson, and Paul D. R. Johnson. "Severe Complications of a 'Brazilian' Bikini Wax." *Clinical Infectious Diseases* 45, no. 3 (2007): e29–e31.

Desruelles, François, Solveig Argeseanu Cunningham, and Dominique Dubois. "Pubic Hair Removal: A Risk Factor for 'Minor' STI Such as Molluscum Contagiosum?" *Sexually Transmitted Infections* 89, no. 3 (2013): 216.

Glass, A. S., H. S. Bagga, G. E. Tasian, P. B. Fisher, C. E. McCulloch, S. D. Blaschko, J. W. McAninch, and B. N. Breyer. "Pubic Hair Grooming Injuries Presenting to U.S. Emergency Departments." *Urology* 80, no. 6 (2012): 1187–91.

Herbenick, D., Schick, V., Reece, M., Sanders, S., and J. D. Fortenberry. "Pubic Hair Removal among Women in the United States: Prevalence, Methods, and Characteristics." *Journal of Sexual Medicine* 7, no. 10 (2010): 3322–30.

G-men, G-spots—They Don't Exist!

Cartwright, Rufus, Susannah Elvy, and Linda Cardozo. "Original Research— Women's Sexual Health: Do Women with Female Ejaculation Have Detrusor Overactivity?" *Journal of Sexual Medicine* 4, no. 6 (2007): 1655–58.

Darling, Carol Anderson, J. Kenneth Davidson Sr., and Colleen Conway-Welch. "Female Ejaculation: Perceived Origins, the Grafenberg Spot/Area, and Sexual Responsiveness." *Archives of Sexual Behavior* 19, no. 1 (1990): 29–47.

Gräfenberg, E. "The Role of Urethra in Female Orgasm." *International Journal of Sexology* 3, no. 3 (1950): 145–48.

Hines, Terence M. "The G-Spot: A Modern Gynecologic Myth." 185, no. 2 (2001): 359–62.

Jannini, E. A., A. Rubio-Casillas, B. Whipple, O. Buisson, B. R. Komisaruk, and S. Brody. "Female Orgasm(s): One, Two, Several." *Journal of Sexual Medicine* 9, no. 4 (2012): 956–65.

Kilchevsky, Amichai, Yoram Vardi, Lior Lowenstein, and Ilan Gruenwald. "Is the Female G-Spot Truly a Distinct Anatomic Entity?" *Journal of Sexual Medicine* 9, no. 3 (2012): 719–26.

Korda, Joanna B., Sue W. Goldstein, and Frank Sommer. "Sexual Medicine History: The History of Female Ejaculation." *Journal of Sexual Medicine* 7, no. 5 (2010): 1965–75.

Ladas, Alice Kahn, Beverly Whipple, and John Perry. *The G Spot and Other Discoveries about Human Sexuality.* New York: Holt, Reinhart and Winston, 1982, 30–85.

Levin, R. J. "Sexual & Relationship Therapy." *Sexual Relationship and Therapy* 18, no. 1 (2003): 117.

Pastor, Zlatko. "[G Spot—Myths and Reality]." *Ceská Gynekologie / Ceská Lékarská Spolecnost J. Ev. Purkyne* 75, no. 3 (2010): 211–17..

Puppo, V. "Anatomy and Physiology of the Clitoris, Vestibular Bulbs, and Labia Minora with a Review of the Female Orgasm and the Prevention of Female Sexual Dysfunction." *Clinical Anatomy* 26, no. 1 (2013): 134–52.

Shafik, Ahmed, Ismail A. Shafik, Olfat El Sibai, and Ali A. Shafik. "An Electro-physiologic Study of Female Ejaculation." *Journal of Sex & Marital Therapy* 35, no. 5 (2009): 337–46.

Zaviacic, M., and R. J. Ablin. "The G-Spot." *American Journal of Obstetrics & Gynecology* 187, no. 2 (2002): 519–20; discusssion 20.

Women Do Not Squirt Like Men

Pastor, Z. "Female Ejaculation Orgasm Vs. Coital Incontinence: A Systematic Review." *Journal of Sexual Medicine* 10, no. 7 (2013): 1682–91.

Wyatt, G. E., S. D. Peters, and D. Guthrie. "Kinsey Revisited, Part I: Comparisons of the Sexual Socialization and Sexual Behavior of White Women over 33 Years." *Archives of Sexual Behavior* 17, no. 3 (1988): 201–39.

Blonds Have More Fun

Grammer, Karl, Bernhard Fink, Anders P. Møller, and Randy Thornhill. "Darwinian Aesthetics: Sexual Selection and the Biology of Beauty." *Biological Reviews of the Cambridge Philosophical Society* 78, no. 3 (2003): 385–407.

Guéguen, Nicolas. "Hair Color and Wages: Waitresses with Blond Hair Have More Fun." *Journal of Socio-Economics* 41, no. 4 (2012): 370–72.

Hazewinkel, Menke H., Ellen T. M. Laan, Mirjam A. G. Sprangers, Guus Fons, Matthé P. M. Burger, and Jan-Paul W. R. Roovers. "Long-Term Sexual Function in Survivors of Vulvar Cancer: A Cross-Sectional Study." *Gynecologic Oncology* 126, no. 1 (2012): 87–92.

Lacelle, Céline, Martine Hébert, Francine Lavoie, Frank Vitaro, and Richard E. Tremblay. "Sexual Health in Women Reporting a History of Child Sexual Abuse." *Child Abuse & Neglect* 36, no. 3 (2012): 247–59.

Rich, Melissa K., and Thomas F. Cash. "The American Image of Beauty: Media Representations of Hair Color for Four Decades." *Sex Roles* 29, no. 1/2 (1993): 113–24.

Nobody Has Pubic Hair These Days

Bercaw-Pratt, Jennifer L., Xiomara M. Santos, Judith Sanchez, Leslie Ayensu-Coker, Denise R. Nebgen, and Jennifer E. Dietrich. "The Incidence, Attitudes and Practices of the Removal of Pubic Hair as a Body Modification." *Journal of Pediatric and Adolescent Gynecology* 25, no. 1 (2012): 12–14.

DeMaria, A. L., and A. B. Berenson. "Prevalence and Correlates of Pubic Hair Grooming among Low-Income Hispanic, Black, and White Women." *Body Image* 10, no. 2 (2013): 226–31.

Dendle, Claire, Sheila Mulvey, Felicity Pyrlis, M. Lindsay Grayson, and Paul D. R. Johnson. "Severe Complications of a 'Brazilian' Bikini Wax." *Clinical Infectious Diseases* 45, no. 3 (2007): e29–e31.

Friedland, Roger. "Looking Through the Bushes: The Disappearance of Pubic Hair." Accessed July 10, 2013. http://www.huffingtonpost.com/roger-friedland/women-pubic-hair_b_875465.html.

Glass, A. S., H. S. Bagga, G. E. Tasian, P. B. Fisher, C. E. McCulloch, S. D. Blaschko, J. W. McAninch, and B. N. Breyer. "Pubic Hair Grooming Injuries Presenting to U.S. Emergency Departments." *Urology* 80, no. 6 (2012): 1187–91.

Herbenick, D., Schick, V., Reece, M., Sanders, S., and J. D. Fortenberry. "Pubic Hair Removal among Women in the United States: Prevalence, Methods, and Characteristics." *Journal of Sexual Medicine* 7, no. 10 (2010): 3322–30.

Little Lost Tampon, Where Did It Go?

Hoffman, B. L., J .O. Schorge, J. I. Schaffer, L. M. Halvorson, K. D. Bradshaw, F. G. Cunningham, and L. E. Calver. "Well Woman Care." *Williams Gynecology*, Second Edition. New York: McGraw-Hill, 2012, 2–32.

A Woman Needs Her Clitoris Stimulated to Have an Orgasm

Herbenick, Debby, Michael Reece, Vanessa Schick, Stephanie A. Sanders, Brian Dodge, and J. Dennis Fortenberry. "Sexual Behaviors, Relationships, and Perceived Health Status among Adult Women in the United States: Results from a National Probability Sample." *Journal of Sexual Medicine* 7 (2010): 277–90.

Holstege, G., J. R. Georgiadis, A. M. Paans, L. C. Meiners, F. H. van der Graaf, and A. A. Reinders. "Brain Activation During Human Male Ejaculation." *Journal of Neuroscience* 23, no. 27 (2003): 9185–93.

Huynh, Hieu Kim, Antoon T. M. Willemsen, and Gert Holstege. "Female Orgasm but Not Male Ejaculation Activates the Pituitary. A Pet-Neuro-Imaging Study." *NeuroImage* 76 (2013): 178–82.

Jannini, E. A., A. Rubio-Casillas, B. Whipple, O. Buisson, B. R. Komisaruk, and S. Brody. "Female Orgasm(s): One, Two, Several." *Journal of Sexual Medicine* 9, no. 4 (2012): 956–65.

King, R., J. Belsky, K. Mah, and Y. Binik. "Are There Different Types of Female Orgasm?" *Archives of Sexual Behavior* 40, no. 5 (2011): 865–75.

Kinsey, Alfred C., ed. *Sexual Behavior in the Human Female.* Philadelphia: Saunders, 1953, 132–73, 346–92, 510–37.

Komisaruk, B. R., N. Wise, E. Frangos, W. C. Liu, K. Allen, and S. Brody. "Women's Clitoris, Vagina, and Cervix Mapped on the Sensory Cortex: FMRI Evidence." *Journal of Sexual Medicine* 8, no. 10 (2011): 2822–30.

Reinisch, J. M., and R. Beasley. *The Kinsey Institute New Report on Sex: What You Must Know to Be Sexually Literate.* New York: St. Martin's Press, 1990.

Waldinger, M. D., G. J. de Lint, A. P. van Gils, F. Masir, E. Lakke, R. S. van Coevorden, and D. H. Schweitzer. "Foot Orgasm Syndrome: A Case Report in a Woman." *Journal of Sexual Medicine* 10, no. 8 (2013): 1926–34.

Buy Our Product for That Clean, Fresh Feeling!

Caliskan, D., N. Subasi, and O. Sarisen. "Vaginal Douching and Associated Factors among Married Women Attending a Family Planning Clinic or a Gynecology Clinic." *European Journal of Obstetrics Gynecology and Reoproductibe Biology* 127, no. 2 (2006): 244–51.

Cottrell, B. H. "An Updated Review of of Evidence to Discourage Douching." no. 1539–0683 (Electronic).

Shaaban, O., Alaa Eldin A. Youssef, Mostafa M. Khodry, and S. A. Mostafa. "Vaginal Douching by Women with Vulvovaginitis and Relation to Reproductive Health Hazards." *BMC Women's Health* 13, no. 1 (2013): 1–6.

Sutton, Madeline Y., Carol Bruce, Maya R. Sternberg, Geraldine McQuillan, Juliette S. Kendrick, Emilia Koumans, and Lauri Markowitz. "Prevalence and Correlates of Vaginal Douching among Women in the United States, 2001–2002." Paper presented at the National STD Prevention Conference, Jacksonville, FL, 2006.

Bigger Breasts Are Less Sensitive

Courtiss, and R. M. Goldwyn. "Breast Sensation before and after Plastic Surgery." *Plastic and Reconstructive Surgery* 58, no. 1 (1976): 1–13.

Tairych G. V., R. Kuzbari, S. Rigel, B. P. Todoroff, B. Schneider, and M. Deutinger. "Normal Cutaneous Sensibility of the Breast." *Plastic and Reconstructive Surgery* 102, no. 3 (1976): 701–4.

That Hole Does Nothing for Me

Bogart, Laura M., Heather Cecil, David A. Wagstaff, Steven D. Pinkerton, and Paul R. Abramson. "Is It 'Sex'?: College Students' Interpretations of Sexual Behavior Terminology." *Journal of Sex Research* 37, no. 2 (2000): 108–16.

Bohlen, Joseph G., James P. Held, Margaret Olwen Sanderson, and Andrew Ahlgren. "The Female Orgasm: Pelvic Contractions." *Archives of Sexual Behavior* 11, no. 5 (1982): 367–86.

Costa, Rui M., and Stuart Brody. "Anxious and Avoidant Attachment, Vibrator

Use, Anal Sex, and Impaired Vaginal Orgasm." *Journal of Sexual Medicine* 8, no. 9 (2011): 2493–500.

————. "Immature Defense Mechanisms Are Associated with Lesser Vaginal Orgasm Consistency and Greater Alcohol Consumption before Sex." *Journal of Sexual Medicine* 7, no. 2 Pt. 1 (2010): 775–86.

Richters, Juliet, Richard de Visser, Chris Rissel, and Anthony Smith. "Sexual Practices at Last Heterosexual Encounter and Occurrence of Orgasm in a National Survey." *Journal of Sex Research* 43, no. 3 (2006): 217–26.

PART III: SEX

Oysters, Chocolate, Bananas . . . Viagra?

Afoakwa, E. O. "Cocoa and Chocolate Consumption—Are There Aphrodisiac and Other Benefits for Human Health?" *South African Journal of Clinical Nutrition* 21, no. 3 (2008): 107–13.

di Tomaso, E., M. Beltramo, and D. Piomelli. "Brain Cannabinoids in Chocolate." *Nature* 382, no. 6593 (1996): 677–78.

Choco GuateMaya. "Cacao: Food for the Gods." http://www.chocoguatemaya .com/origin_eng.php.

Engler, Mary B., Marguerite M. Engler, Chung Y. Chen, Mary J. Malloy, Amanda Browne, Elisa Y. Chiu, Ho-Kyung Kwak, Paul Milbury, Steven M. Paul, Jeffrey Blumberg, and Michele L. Mietus-Snyder. "Flavonoid-Rich Dark Chocolate Improves Endothelial Function and Increases Plasma Epicatechin Concentrations in Healthy Adults." *Journal of the American College of Nutrition* 23, no. 3 (2004): 197–204.

Malviya, N., S. Jain, V. B. Gupta, and S. Vyas. "Recent Studies on Aphrodisiac Herbs for the Management of Male Sexual Dysfunction—A Review." *Acta Poloniae Pharmaceutica* 68, no. 1 (2011): 3–8.

Patel, D. K., R. Kumar, S. K. Prasad, and S. Hemalatha. "Pharmacologically Screened Aphrodisiac Plant—a Review of Current Scientific Literature." *Asian Pacific Journal of Tropical Biomedicine* 1, no. 1, Supplement (2011): S131–S38.

Sudano, I., A. J. Flammer, S. Roas, F. Enseleit, F. Ruschitzka, R. Corti, and G. Noll. "Cocoa, Blood Pressure, and Vascular Function." *Current Hypertension Reports* 14, no. 4 (2012): 279–84.

Vlachopoulos, Charalambos, Nikolaos Alexopoulos, and Christodoulos Stefanadis. "Effect of Dark Chocolate on Arterial Function in Healthy Individuals: Cocoa Instead of Ambrosia?" *Current Hypertension Reports* 8, no. 3 (2006): 205–11.

Don't Put *That* in *There*!

Aggrawal, A. "A New Classification of Zoophilia." *Journal of Forensic and Legal Medicine* 18, no. 2 (2011): 73–78.

Benson, Paul A. S., Amy B. Middleman, and Mary M. Torchia. "Patient

Information: Adolescent Sexuality (Beyond the Basics)." Up to Date, http://www.uptodate.com/contents/adolescent-sexuality-beyond-the-basics.

Dreben, R. E., M. Knight, and M. A. Sindhian. *Stuck Up! 100 Objects Inserted and Ingested in Places They Shouldn't Be.* New York: St. Martin's Press, 2011.

Goldberg, J. E., and S. R. Steele. "Rectal Foreign Bodies." *Surgical Clinics of North America* 90, no. 1 (2010): 173–84, Table of Contents.

Kirov, G. K., J. E. Losanoff, and K. T. Kjossev. "Zoophilia: A Rare Cause of Traumatic Injury to the Rectum." *Injury* 33, no. 4 (2002): 367–68.

Lake, J. P., R. Essani, P. Petrone, A. M. Kaiser, J. Asensio, and R. W. Beart Jr. "Management of Retained Colorectal Foreign Bodies: Predictors of Operative Intervention." *Diseases of the Colon & Rectum* 47, no. 10 (2004): 1694–98.

Reinisch, J. M., and R. Beasley. "America Fails Sex Information Test." *The Kinsey Institute New Report on Sex,* edited by Debra Kent. New York: St. Martin's Press, 1990, 7–8.

Zequi Sde, C., G. C. Guimaraes, F. P. da Fonseca, U. Ferreira, W. E. de Matheus, L. O. Reis, G. A. Aita, S. Glina, V. S. Fanni, M. D. Perez, L. R. Guidoni, V. Ortiz, L. Nogueira, L. C. de Almeida Rocha, G. Cuck, W. H. da Costa, R. R. Moniz, J. H. Dantas Jr., F. A. Soares, and A. Lopes. "Sex with Animals (Swa): Behavioral Characteristics and Possible Association with Penile Cancer. A Multicenter Study." *Journal of Sexual Medicine* 9, no. 7 (2012): 1860–67.

It Will Really Turn a Woman On If You Do the Laundry

Amato, Paul R., A. Booth, D. R. Johnson, and S. J. Rogers. *Alone Together: How Marriage in America Is Changing.* Boston, MA: Harvard University Press, 2007, 1–70.

Chethik, N. *Voicemale: What Husbands Really Think About Their Marriages, Their Wives, Sex, Housework, and Commitment.* New York: Simon and Schuster, 2006, 97–203.

Gager, Constance T., and Scott T. Yabiku. "Who Has the Time? The Relationship between Household Labor Time and Sexual Frequency." *Journal of Family Issues* 31, no. 2 (2009): 135–63.

Hook, Jennifer L. "Care in Context: Men's Unpaid Work in 20 Countries, 1965–2003." *American Sociological Review* 71, no. 4 (2006): 639–60.

Kornrich, Sabino, Julie Brines, and Katrina Leupp. "Egalitarianism, Housework, and Sexual Frequency in Marriage." *American Sociological Review* 78, no. 1 (2013): 26–50.

Witting, Katarina, Pekka Santtila, Markus Varjonen, Patrick Jern, Ada Johansson, Bettina von der Pahlen, and Kenneth Sandnabba. "Female Sexual Dysfunction, Sexual Distress, and Compatibility with Partner." *Journal of Sexual Medicine* 5, no. 11 (2008): 2587–99.

Don't Leave Your Socks On!

Brain, A. E. "Keep Your Socks On." http://aebrain.blogspot.com/2005/07/keep-your-socks-on.html.

Georgiadis, Janniko R., Rudie Kortekaas, Rutger Kuipers, Arie Nieuwenburg, Jan

Pruim, A. A. T. Simone Reinders, and Gert Holstege. "Regional Cerebral Blood Flow Changes Associated with Clitorally Induced Orgasm in Healthy Women." *European Journal of Neuroscience* 24, no. 11 (2006): 3305–16.

Holstege, G., J. R. Georgiadis, A. M. Paans, L. C. Meiners, F. H. van der Graaf, and A. A. Reinders. "Brain Activation During Human Male Ejaculation." *Journal of Neuroscience* 23, no. 27 (2003): 9185–93.

Huynh, Hieu Kim, Antoon T. M. Willemsen, and Gert Holstege. "Female Orgasm but Not Male Ejaculation Activates the Pituitary. A Pet-Neuro-Imaging Study." *NeuroImage* 76 (2013): 178–82.

Kent, William. "Why You Should Keep Your Socks On in Bed." Elite Daily, http://elitedaily.com/dating/sex/wearing-socks-30-orgasm/.

Lose Weight Fast! Have Sex!

Bohlen, J. G., J. P. Held, M. O. Sanderson, and R. P. Patterson. "Heart Rate, Rate-Pressure Product, and Oxygen Uptake During Four Sexual Activities." *Archives of Internal Medicine* 144, no. 9 (1984): 1745–48.

Chen, X., Q. Zhang, and X. Tan. "Cardiovascular Effects of Sexual Activity." *Indian Journal of Medical Research* 130, no. 6 (2009): 681–88.

Levine, G. N., E. E. Steinke, F. G. Bakaeen, B. Bozkurt, M. D. Cheitlin, J. B. Conti, E. Foster, T. Jaarsma, R. A. Kloner, R. A. Lange, S. T. Lindau, B. J. Maron, D. K. Moser, E. M. Ohman, A. D. Seftel, and W. J. Stewart. "Sexual Activity and Cardiovascular Disease: A Scientific Statement from the American Heart Association." *Circulation* 125, no. 8 (2012): 1058–72.

Lindau, S. T., E. Abramsohn, K. Gosch, K. Wroblewski, E. S. Spatz, P. S. Chan, J. Spertus, and H. M. Krumholz. "Patterns and Loss of Sexual Activity in the Year Following Hospitalization for Acute Myocardial Infarction (a United States National Multisite Observational Study)." *American Journal of Cardiology* 109, no. 10 (2012): 1439–44.

Waldinger, M. D., P. Quinn, M. Dilleen, R. Mundayat, D. H. Schweitzer, and M. Boolell. "A Multinational Population Survey of Intravaginal Ejaculation Latency Time." *Journal of Sexual Medicine* 2, no. 4 (2005): 492–97.

World Health Organization. "What Is Moderate-Intensity and Vigorous-Intensity Physical Activity?" http://www.who.int/dietphysicalactivity/physical_activity_intensity/en/.

To Be or Not to Be . . . Pierced

Anderson, W. R., D. J. Summerton, D. M. Sharma, and S. A. Holmes. "The Urologist's Guide to Genital Piercing." *BJU International* 91, no. 3 (2003): 245–51.

Buhrich, Neil. "The Association of Erotic Piercing with Homosexuality, Sadomasochism, Bondage, Fetishism, and Tattoos." *Archives of Sexual Behavior* 12, no. 2 (1983): 167–71.

Catania, Lucrezia, Omar Abdulcadir, Vincenzo Puppo, Jole Baldaro Verde, Jasmine Abdulcadir, and Dalmar Abdulcadir. "Pleasure and Orgasm in Women with Female Genital Mutilation/Cutting (FGM/C)." *Journal of Sexual Medicine* 4, no. 6 (2007): 1666–78.

Miller, Leslie, and Monica Edenholm. "Genital Piercing to Enhance Sexual Satisfaction." *Obstetrics & Gynecology* 93, no. 5 Pt. 2 (1999): 837.

Millner, V. S., B. H. Eichold, 2nd, T. H. Sharpe, and S. C. Lynn Jr. "First Glimpse of the Functional Benefits of Clitoral Hood Piercings." *American Journal of Obstetrics & Gynecology* 193, no. 3 Pt. 1 (2005): 675–76.

Skegg, K., S. Nada-Raja, C. Paul, and D. C. Skegg. "Body Piercing, Personality, and Sexual Behavior." *Archives of Sexual Behavior* 36, no. 1 (2007): 47–54.

Young, C., M. L. Armstrong, A. E. Roberts, I. Mello, and E. Angel. "A Triad of Evidence for Care of Women with Genital Piercings." *Journal of the American Academy of Nurse Practitioners* 22, no. 2 (2010): 70–80.

Methuselah Had Sex Ten Times a Day

Davey Smith, G., S. Frankel, and J. Yarnell. "Sex and Death: Are They Related? Findings from the Caerphilly Cohort Study." *BMJ (Clinical Research Ed.)* 315, no. 7123 (1997): 1641–44.

Lindau, S. T., E. Abramsohn, K. Gosch, K. Wroblewski, E. S. Spatz, P. S. Chan, J. Spertus, and H. M. Krumholz. "Patterns and Loss of Sexual Activity in the Year Following Hospitalization for Acute Myocardial Infarction (a United States National Multisite Observational Study)." *American Journal of Cardiology* 109, no. 10 (2012): 1439–44.

Onder, G., B. W. Penninx, J. M. Guralnik, H. Jones, L. P. Fried, M. Pahor, and J. D. Williamson. "Sexual Satisfaction and Risk of Disability in Older Women." *Journal of Clinical Psychiatry* 64, no. 10 (2003): 1177–82.

Palmore, E. B. "Predictors of the Longevity Difference: A 25-Year Follow-Up." *Gerontologist* 22, no. 6 (1982): 513–18.

Squeezing Breasts Is All Fun and Games

Levin, Roy, and Cindy Meston. "Nipple/Breast Stimulation and Sexual Arousal in Young Men and Women." *Journal of Sexual Medicine* 3, no. 3 (2006): 450–54.

Wiseman, Bryony S., and Zena Werb. "Stromal Effects on Mammary Gland Development and Breast Cancer." *Science* 296, no. 5570 (2002): 1046–49.

Get Out of Those Pajamas!

ABC News. "The American Sex Survey: A Peek beneath the Sheets." 10/21/04.

Molloy, H. F., E. LaMont-Gregory, C. Idzikowski, and T. J. Ryan. "Overheating in Bed as an Important Factor in Many Common Dermatoses." *International Journal of Dermatology* 32, no. 9 (1993): 668–72.

PR Newswire. "National Sleep Survey Pulls Back the Covers on How We Dose and Dream." http://www.prnewswire.com/news-releases/national-sleep-survey-pulls-back-the-covers-on-how-we-doze-and-dream-184798691.html.

Can't Buy Me Love

Barrientos, Jaime E., and Dario Páez. "Psychosocial Variables of Sexual Satisfaction in Chile." *Journal of Sex & Marital Therapy* 32, no. 5 (2006): 351–68.

Blanchflower, D. G., and A. J. Oswald. "Money, Sex, and Happiness: An Empirical Study." *Scandinavian Journal of Economics* 106, no. 3 (2004): 393–415.

Hawton, K., D. Gath, and A. Day. "Sexual Function in a Community Sample of Middle-Aged Women with Partners: Effects of Age, Marital, Socioeconomic, Psychiatric, Gynecological, and Menopausal Factors." *Archives of Sexual Behavior* 23, no. 4 (1994): 375–95.

Nettle, D., and T. V. Pollet. "Natural Selection on Male Wealth in Humans." *American Naturalist* 172, no. 5 (2008): 658–66.

Pollet, Thomas V., and Daniel Nettle. "Partner Wealth Predicts Self-Reported Orgasm Frequency in a Sample of Chinese Women." *Evolution and Human Behavior* 30, no. 2 (2009): 146–51.

Television Makes You Oversexed

Alexander, B. "When the Only Connections in Bed Are Wireless." NBCNews.com, http://www.nbcnews.com/id/23749828/ns/health-sexual_health/t/when-only-connections-bed-are-wireless/#.Uc2w2j5ARYw.

"American Academy of Pediatrics. Policy Statement—Sexuality, Contraception, and the Media." *Pediatrics* 126, no. 3 (2010): 576–82.

Brunborg, Geir Scott, Rune Aune Mentzoni, Helge Molde, Helga Myrseth, Knut Joachim Mår Skouverøe, Bjørn Bjorvatn, and Ståle Pallesen. "The Relationship between Media Use in the Bedroom, Sleep Habits and Symptoms of Insomnia." *Journal of Sleep Research* 20, no. 4 (2011): 569–75.

Kunkel, D., K. M. Cope, and C. Colvin. *Sexual Messages on Family Hour Television: Content and Context.* Menlo Park, CA: Kaiser Family Foundation, 1996.

Kunkel, D., K. Eyal, E. Donnerstein, K. M. Farrar, E. Biely, and V. Rideout. "Sexual Socialization Messages on Entertainment Television: Comparing Content Trends 1997–2002." *Media Psychology* 9, no. 3 (2007): 595–622.

Kunkel, D., K. Eyal, K. Finnerty, E. Biely, and E. Donnerstein. *Sex on Tv 4: A Biennial Report to the Kaiser Family Foundation.* Menlo Park, CA: Kaiser Family Foundation, 2005.

Leibovich, L. "Turn Off the Tube, Have More Sex." Salon Media Group, Inc., http://www.salon.com/2006/01/17/sex_tv/.

National Sleep Foundation. "Sleep in America 2010." Washington, D.C., 2010. http://www.sleepfoundation.org/.

Sidner, S. "Less Sex, More Tv Idea Aired in India." CNN, http://www.cnn.com/2009/WORLD/asiapcf/08/13/sex.or.tv/.

Ward, M. "Contributions of Entertainment Television to Adolescents' Sexual Attitudes and Expectations: The Role of Viewing Amount Versus Viewer Involvement." *Journal of Sex Research* 36, no. 3 (1999): 237–49.

It's Only a Matter of Time Until a Man Cheats

Allen, Elizabeth S., David C. Atkins, Donald H. Baucom, Douglas K. Snyder, Kristina Coop Gordon, and Shirley P. Glass. "Intrapersonal, Interpersonal, and Contextual Factors in Engaging in and Responding to Extramarital Involvement." *Clinical Psychology: Science and Practice* 12, no. 2 (2005): 101–30.

Barta, William D., and Susan M. Kiene. "Motivations for Infidelity in Heterosexual Dating Couples: The Roles of Gender, Personality Differences, and Sociosexual Orientation." *Journal of Social and Personal Relationships* 22, no. 3 (2005): 339–60.

Burdette, Amy M., Christopher G. Ellison, Darren E. Sherkat, and Kurt A. Gore. "Are There Religious Variations in Marital Infidelity?" *Journal of Family Issues* 28, no. 12 (2007): 1553–81.

Jamison, Paul L., and Paul H. Gebhard. "Penis Size Increase between Flaccid and Erect States: An Analysis of the Kinsey Data." *Journal of Sex Research* 24 (1988): 177–83.

Mark, K. P., E. Janssen, and R. R. Milhausen. "Infidelity in Heterosexual Couples: Demographic, Interpersonal, and Personality-Related Predictors of Extradyadic Sex." *Archives of Sexual Behavior* 40, no. 5 (2011): 971–82.

Mattingly, Brent A., Karen Wilson, Eddie M. Clark, Amanda W. Bequette, and Daniel J. Weidler. "Foggy Faithfulness: Relationship Quality, Religiosity, and the Perceptions of Dating Infidelity Scale in an Adult Sample." *Journal of Family Issues* 31, no. 11 (2010): 1465–80.

Wessells, Hunter, Tom F. Lue, and Jack W. McAninch. "Penile Length in the Flaccid and Erect States: Guidelines for Penile Augmentation." *Journal of Urology* 156, no. 3 (1996): 995–97.

Wiederman, Michael W. "Extramarital Sex: Prevalence and Correlates in a National Survey." *Journal of Sex Research* 34, no. 2 (1997): 167–74.

There's a Ten-Year Difference in Sexual Peaks

Herbenick, D., Reece, M., Schick, V., Sanders, S., Dodge, B., and J. D. Fortenberry. "Sexual Behavior in the United States: Results from a National Probability Sample of Men and Women Ages 14–94." *Journal of Sexual Medicine* 7 (2010): 255–65.

Only Teenagers Come Too Soon

Laumann, E. O., A. Paik, and R. C. Rosen. "Sexual Dysfunction in the United States: Prevalence and Predictors." *JAMA* 281, no. 6 (1999): 537–44.

Rowland, D., C. G. McMahon, C. Abdo, J. Chen, E. Jannini, M. D. Waldinger, and

T. Y. Ahn. "Disorders of Orgasm and Ejaculation in Men." *Journal of Sexual Medicine* 7, no. 4 Pt. 2 (2010): 1668–86.

Watching Porn Is a Guy Thing

Buzzell, Timothy. "Demographic Characteristics of Persons Using Pornography in Three Technological Contexts." *Sexuality & Culture* 9, no. 1 (2005): 28–48.

Cooper, Alvin, Coralie R. Scherer, Sylvain C. Boies, and Barry L. Gordon. "Sexuality on the Internet: From Sexual Exploration to Pathological Expression." *Professional Psychology: Research and Practice* 30, no. 2 (1999): 154–64.

Weinberg, M. S., C. J. Williams, S. Kleiner, and Y. Irizarry. "Pornography, Normalization, and Empowerment." *Archives of Sexual Behavior* 39, no. 6 (2010): 1389–401.

Wolak, Janis, Kimberly Mitchell, and David Finkelhor. "Unwanted and Wanted Exposure to Online Pornography in a National Sample of Youth Internet Users." *Pediatrics* 119, no. 2 (2007): 247–57.

Wright, P. J. "U.S. Males and Pornography, 1973–2010: Consumption, Predictors, Correlates." *Journal of Sex Research* 50, no. 1 (2013): 60–71.

Men Want It More. Way, Way More.

Herbenick, Debby, Michael Reece, Vanessa Schick, Stephanie A. Sanders, Brian Dodge, and J. Dennis Fortenberry. "Sexual Behavior in the United States: Results from a National Probability Sample of Men and Women Ages 14–94." *Journal of Sexual Medicine* 7 (2010): 255–65.

The Kinsey Institute. "The Kinsey Institute—Sexuality Information Links—Faq [Related Resources]." http://www.kinseyinstitute.org/resources/FAQ.html.

Laumann, Edward O. *The Social Organization of Sexuality: Sexual Practices in the United States.* Chicago, IL: University of Chicago Press, 1994, 86–111.

I Can't Do That . . . It Will Give Me Hemorrhoids

Janicke, D. M., and M. R. Pundt. "Anorectal disorders." *Emergency Medical Clinics of North America,*14, no. 4 (1996): 757–88.

You'll Never Go Gray . . . Down There

Haga, K., K. Terazawa, T. Takatori, H. Mikami, and T. Tsukamoto. "[Age Estimation by Appearance of Gray Hair in Pubic Hair]." *Nihon Hoigaku Zasshi* 49, no. 1 (1995): 20–25.

Let's Play Back Door, Front Door, Back Door . . .

Cherpes, T. L., Sharon L. Hillier, Leslie A. Meyn, James L. Busch, Marijane A. Busch, and M. A. Krohn. "A Delicate Balance: Risk Factors for Acquisition of Bacterial Vaginosis Include Sexual Activity, Absence of Hydrogen Peroxide-Producing Lactobacilli, Black Race, and Positive Herpes Simplex Virus Type 2 Serology." *Sexually Transmitted Diseases* 35, no. 1 (2008): 78–83.

Married People Don't Play—with Themselves!

Herbenick, Debby, Michael Reece, Vanessa Schick, Stephanie A. Sanders, Brian Dodge, and J. Dennis Fortenberry. "Sexual Behavior in the United States: Results from a National Probability Sample of Men and Women Ages 14–94." *Journal of Sexual Medicine* 7 (2010): 255–65.

Janus, S. *The Janus Report on Sexual Behavior.* New York: John Wiley & Sons, 1993, 53–102.

Pinkerton, Steven D., Laura M. Bogart, Heather Cecil, and Paul R. Abramson. "Factors Associated with Masturbation in Collegiate Sample." *Journal of Psychology & Human Sexuality* 14, no. 2–3 (2002): 103–21.

Women Are Turned Off by Sweaty, Stinky Men

Wyart, C., Wallace W. Webster, Jonathan H. Webster, Sarah R. Chen, Andrew Wilson Sr., Rehan M. McClary, Noam Khan, and N. Sobel. "Smelling a Single Component of Male Sweat Alters Levels of Cortisol in Women." *Journal of Neuroscience* 27, no. 6 (2007): 1261–65.

When in Doubt, Double-Bag It

Blankenship, K. M. Brook S. West, Trace S. West, Monica R. Kershaw, and M. R. Biradavolu. "Power, Community Mobilization, and Condom Use Practices among Female Sex Workers in Andhra Pradesh, India." *AIDS,* supplement 5 (2008): 109–16.

Rugpao, S., C. Beyrer, S. Tovanabutra, C. Natpratan, K. E. Nelson, D. D. Celentano, and C. Khamboonruang. "Multiple Condom Use and Decreased Condom Breakage and Slippage in Thailand." *Journal of Acquired Immune Deficiency Syndromes and Human Retrovirology* 14, no. 2 (1997): 169–73.

Rugpao, S., S. Tovanabutra, C. Tovanabutra, C. Beyrer, D. Nuntakuang, Y. Yutabootr, T. Vongchak, M. A. de Boer, D. D. Celentano, and K. E. Nelson. "Multiple Condom Use in Commercial Sex in Lamphun Province, Thailand: A Community-Generated Std/Hiv Prevention Strategy." *Sexually Transmitted Diseases* 24, no. 9 (1997): 546–49.

The Stiff Has a Stiff

Dead Serious News. "Dead Man in Mortuary Impregnates Woman." http://www.deadseriousnews.com/dead-man-in-mortuary-impregnates-woman/.

Did She or Didn't She? Faking It for Beginners

Huynh, Hieu Kim, Antoon T. M. Willemsen, and Gert Holstege. "Female Orgasm but Not Male Ejaculation Activates the Pituitary. A Pet-Neuro-Imaging Study." *NeuroImage* 76 (2013): 178–82.

Muehlenhard, C. L., and S. K. Shippee. (2010). "Men's and women's reports of pretending orgasm." *Journal of Sex Research* 47, no. 6 (2010): 552–67.

Only Men Have Wet Dreams

Henton, C. L. (1976). "Nocturnal Orgasm in College Women: Its Relation to Dreams and Anxiety Associated with Sexual Factors." *Journal of Genetic Psychology* 129, no. 2 (1976): 245–51.

Masturbation Will Make You Go Blind

Ashworth, Michael. "Do Kellogg's Corn Flakes Help Control Masturbation?" PsychCentral, http://psychcentral.com/lib/2007/do-kelloggs-corn-flakes-help-control-masturbation/.

———. "Does Masturbation Cause Blindness?" PsychCentral, http://psychcentral.com/lib/2007/does-masturbation-cause-blindness/.

Auteri, Steph. "5 Bogus Masturbation Myths." YourTango, http://www.yourtango.com/201055179/5-bogus-masturbation-myths.

Dr. V. "Doin' It with Dr. V: Masturbation Myths." TheFrisky, http://www.thefrisky.com/post/246-doin-it-with-dr-v-masturbation-myths/.

Macintyre, Ben. "Birthday of One Mighty Flake . . . And a Cereal Too." *The Times,* http://www.timesonline.co.uk/tol/news/world/us_and_americas/article732027.ece.

Shaw, Jim. "Masturbation Myths." 4-Men.org, http://www.4-men.org/myths-about-masturbation.html.

Silverberg, Cory. "100 Years of Fighting Masturbation, One Spoonful at a Time." About.com, http://sexuality.about.com/b/2006/02/20/100-years-of-fighting-masturbation-one-spoonful-at-a-time.htm.

Witmer, Denise. "Masturbation Myths." About.com, http://parentingteens.about.com/od/masterbationmyths/a/masterbation.htm.

Sex Can Give You a Heart Attack

BBC News. "BBC News—Heart attack survivors fear sex." Accessed June 24, 2013. http://news.bbc.co.uk/2/hi/8696801.stm.

Hall, S. A., Shakelton R., Rosen R. C., and A. B. Araujo. "Sexual Activity, Erectile Dysfunction, and Incident Cardiovascular Events." *American Journal of Cardiology* 105, no. 2 (2010): 192–97.

Hendrick, Bill. "More Sex Could Mean Less Heart Risk." Accessed October 6, 2010. http://www.webmd.com/heart-disease/news/20100121/more-sex-could-mean-less-heart-risk.

Silverburg, Cory. "Heart Attack During Sex—How Common Are Heart Attacks During Sex." Accessed October 6, 2010. http://sexuality.about.com/od/sexualhealthqanda/f/heart_attack_during_sex.htm.

———. "Sex and Heart Disease Myths—Myths Sexual Activity and Heart Disease." Accessed October 6, 2010. http://sexuality.about.com/od/sexual healthqanda/a/myths_about_sex_and_heart_disease_attack.htm.

———. "Sex After a Heart Attack—Resuming Sex After a Heart Attack." Accessed October 6, 2010. http://sexuality.about.com/od/sexualhealthqanda/a/sex_after_heart_attack.htm.

Telegraph.co.uk. "Having sex twice a week 'reduces chance of heart attack by half.'" Accessed October 6, 2010. http://www.telegraph.co.uk/health/healthnews/6950548/Having-sex-twice-a-week-reduces-chance-of-heart-attack-by-half.htm.

WebMD. Web site Title. Accessed June 24, 2013. http://www.webmd.com/heart-disease/features/sex-after-a-heart-attack.

PART IV: GETTING PREGNANT

You Can't Get Pregnant During Your Period

Fertility Friend. "All About Ovulation." http://www.fertilityfriend.com/Faqs/Ovulation.html.

KidsHealth. "Can a Girl Get Pregnant If She Has Sex During Her Period?" Nemours Foundation, http://kidshealth.org/teen/expert/sex_health/sex_during_period.html.

If a Woman Has an Orgasm, It Is More Likely She Will Get Pregnant

Beck, J. R. "How Do the Spermatozoa Enter the Uterus?" *American Journal of Obstetrics & Gynecology* 4, no. 7 (1874): 350–91.

Levin, Roy J. "Can the Controversy About the Putative Role of the Human Female Orgasm in Sperm Transport Be Settled with Our Current Physiological Knowledge of Coitus?" *Journal of Sexual Medicine* 8, no. 6 (2011): 1566–78.

———. "The Physiology of Sexual Arousal in the Human Female: A Recreational and Procreational Synthesis." *Archives of Sexual Behavior* 31, no. 5 (2002): 405–11.

———. "Sexual Arousal—Its Physiological Roles in Human Reproduction." *Annual Review of Sex Research* 16 (2005): 154–89.

You Can't Get Pregnant If It Was a Rape

Holmes, M. M., H. S. Resnick, D. G. Kilpatrick, and C. L. Best "Rape-related pregnancy: estimates and descriptive characteristics from a national sample of women." *American Journal of Obstetrics & Gynecology*, 175, no. 2 (1996): 320–24; discussion 324–325.

The Pill Will Make You Fat

Gallo, M. F., L. M. Lopez, D. A. Grimes, K. F. Schulz, and F. M. Helmerhorst. "Combination Contraceptives: Effects on Weight." *Cochrane Database of Systematic Reviews*, no. 9 (2011): CD003987.

Warholm, L., K. R. Petersen, and P. Ravn. "Combined Oral Contraceptives' Influence on Weight, Body Composition, Height, and Bone Mineral Density in Girls Younger Than 18 Years: A Systematic Review." *European Journal of Contraception and Reproductive Health Care* 17, no. 4 (2012): 245–53.

Birth Control Pills Don't Work as Well If You're on Antibiotics

Burroughs, K. E., and M. L. Chambliss. "Antibiotics and Oral Contraceptive Failure." *Archives of Family Medicine* 9 (2000): 81–82.

Helms, S. E., D. L. Bredle, J. Zajic, D. Jarjoura, R. T. Brodell, and I Krishnarao. "Oral contraceptive failure rates and oral antibiotics." *Journal of the American Academy of Dermatology* 36 (1997): 705–10.

If You Put on the Pounds, Birth Control Pills Won't Work

Dinger, J. C., M. Cronin, S. Mohner, I. Schellschmidt, T. D. Minh, and C. Westhoff. "Oral Contraceptive Effectiveness According to Body Mass Index, Weight, Age, and Other Factors." *American Journal of Obstetrics & Gynecology* 201, no. 3 (2009): 263 e1–9.

Holt, V. L., K. L. Cushing-Haugen, and J. R. Daling. "Body Weight and Risk of Oral Contraceptive Failure." *Obstetrics & Gynecology* 99, no. 5 Pt. 1 (2002): 820–27.

Westhoff, C. L., A. H. Torgal, E. R. Mayeda, F. Z. Stanczyk, J. P. Lerner, E. K. Benn, and M. Paik. "Ovarian Suppression in Normal-Weight and Obese Women During Oral Contraceptive Use: A Randomized Controlled Trial." *Obstetrics & Gynecology* 116, no. 2 Pt. 1 (2010): 275–83.

IUDs Are Horrible!

Cramer, D. W., et al. "Tubal Infertility and the Intrauterine Device." *New England Journal of Medicine* 312, no. 15 (1985): 941–47.

Daling, J. R., N. S. Weiss, B. J. Metch, W. H. Chow, R. M. Soderstrom, D. E. Moore, L. R. Spadoni, and B. V. Stadel. "Primary Tubal Infertility in Relation to the

Use of an Intrauterine Device." *New England Journal of Medicine* 312, no. 15 (1985): 937–41.

Datey, S., L. N. Gaur, and B. N. Saxena. "Vaginal Bleeding Patterns of Women Using Different Contraceptive Methods (Implants, Injectables, Iuds, Oral Pills)—an Indian Experience. An Icmr Task Force Study. Indian Council of Medical Research." *Contraception* 51, no. 3 (1995): 155–65.

Hubacher, D., R. Lara-Ricalde, D. J. Taylor, F. Guerra-Infante, and R. Guzman-Rodriguez. "Use of Copper Intrauterine Devices and the Risk of Tubal Infertility among Nulligravid Women." *New England Journal of Medicine* 345, no. 8 (2001): 561–67.

Lee, N. C., G. L. Rubin, and R. Borucki. "The Intrauterine Device and Pelvic Inflammatory Disease Revisited: New Results from the Women's Health Study." *Obstetrics & Gynecology* 72, no. 1 (1988): 1–6.

Lee, N. C., G. L. Rubin, H. W. Ory, and R. T. Burkman. "Type of Intrauterine Device and the Risk of Pelvic Inflammatory Disease." *Obstetrics & Gynecology* 62, no. 1 (1983): 1–6.

Meirik, O. "Intrauterine Devices—Upper and Lower Genital Tract Infections." *Contraception* 75, no. 6 Supplement (2007): S41–7.

Moreau, C., J. Trussell, G. Rodriguez, N. Bajos, and J. Bouyer. "Contraceptive Failure Rates in France: Results from a Population-Based Survey." *Human Reproduction* 22, no. 9 (2007): 2422–27.

Segal, S. J., F. Alvarez-Sanchez, C. A. Adejuwon, V. Brache de Mejia, P. Leon, and A. Faundes. "Absence of Chorionic Gonadotropin in Sera of Women Who Use Intrauterine Devices." *Fertility and Sterility* 44, no. 2 (1985): 214–18.

Sivin, I., and I. Batar. "State-of-the-Art of Non-Hormonal Methods of Contraception: Iii. Intrauterine Devices." *European Journal of Contraception and Reproductive Health Care* 15, no. 2 (2010): 96–112.

Skjeldestad, F., and H. Bratt. "Fertility after Complicated and Non-Complicated Use of Iuds. A Controlled Prospective Study." *Advances in Contraception* 4, no. 3 (1988): 179–84.

Tietze, C. "Evaluation of Intrauterine Devices: Ninth Progress Report of the Cooperative Statistical Program." *Studies in Family Planning*, no. 55 (1970): 1–40.

Wilcox, A. J., C. R. Weinberg, R. E. Wehmann, E. G. Armstrong, R. E. Canfield, and B. C. Nisula. "Measuring Early Pregnancy Loss: Laboratory and Field Methods." *Fertility and Sterility* 44, no. 3 (1985): 366–74.

Want a Baby Girl? Turn This Way, Bend That Way.

Gray, R. H. Natural family planning and sex selection: fact or fiction? *American Journal of Obstetrics & Gynecology,* 165, no. 6 Pt. 2 (1991): 1982–84.

Mossman, J. A., J. Slate, T. R. Birkhead, H. D. Moore, and A. A. Pacey. Sperm speed is associated with sex bias of siblings in a human population. *Asian Journal of Andrology*, 15, no. 1 (2013): 152–54. doi: 10.1038/aja.2012.109.

You Can't Get Pregnant If . . .

KidsHealth. "Birth Control Pill." Accessed June 24, 2013. http://www.kidshealth .org/teen/expert/sex_health/sex_during_period.html.

KidsHealth. "Can a Girl Get Pregnant if She Has Sex During Her Period?" Accessed May 20, 2008. http://www.kidshealth.org/PageManager.jsp ?dn=familydoctor&lic=44&cat_id=20015&article_set=20406&ps=209.

KidsHealth. "Withdrawal." Accessed May 21, 2008. http://www.kidshealth.org/ PageManager.jsp?dn=familydoctor&article_set=10581&lic=44&cat _id=20018.

National Campaign to Prevent Teen and Unplanned Pregnancy. Fact Sheet. Accessed June 11, 2008. http://www.teenpregnancy.org/resources/reading/ pdf/myths.pdf.

Planned Parenthood of North Texas. "Birth Control." Accessed June 11, 2008. http://www.ppnt.org/sexual-health/birth-control/birth-control.html.

Poland M. L., K. S. Moghissi, P. T. Giblin, J. W. Ager, and J. M. Olson. "Variation of semen measures within normal men." *Fertility and Sterility* 44 (1985): 396–400.

PART V: SEXUALLY TRANSMITTED INFECTIONS

You Didn't Get That STD from Sex

Hedgepeth, Albert William, Jr. "Can You Get an STD from a Toilet Seat?" http:// www.ehow.com/video_4872259_can-std-toilet-seat_.html.

Centers for Disease Control and Prevention. "Hiv Transmission." http://www.cdc .gov/hiv/resources/qa/transmission.htm.

Dayan, L. "Transmission of Neisseria Gonorrhoeae from a Toilet Seat." *Sexually Transmitted Infections* 80, no. 4 (2004): 327.

Herpes Resource Center. "Herpes Myths Vs. Facts." http://herpesresourcecenter .com/mvf.html.

Peiperl, Laurence. "Va National Hiv/Aids Web site: Frequently Asked Questions." http://www.hiv.va.gov/patient/faqs/life-expectancy-with-HIV.asp.

But What About Crabs? I Know You Can Get Those from the Toilet Seat!

Allyson, Dionne. "What Stds Can You Get from a Toilet Seat." http://www.ehow .com/video_4872259_can-std-toilet-seat_.html.

WebMD. "What Can You Catch in Restrooms?". http://www.webmd.com/balance/
features/what-can-you-catch-in-restrooms?page=2.

Oral Sex Is Totally Safe

Centers for Disease Control and Prevention. "Hiv Transmission." http://www.cdc
.gov/hiv/resources/qa/transmission.htm.
Herpes Resource Center. "Herpes Myths Vs. Facts." http://herpesresourcecenter
.com/mvf.html.
"Hotline: Can You Get an Std from Oral Sex?". http://www.stdtestexpress.com/
blog/hotline-can-you-get-an-std-from-oral-sex/.
Peiperl, Laurence. "Va National Hiv/Aids Web site: Frequently Asked Questions."
http://www.hiv.va.gov/patient/faqs/life-expectancy-with-HIV.asp.

Condoms Will Protect You from Anything

Steiner, M. J., and W. Cates Jr. "Condoms and Sexually-Transmitted Infections."
New England Journal of Medicine 354, no. 25 (2006): 2642–43.
Wald, Anna, Andria G. M. Langenberg, Elizabeth Krantz, John M. Douglas Jr., H.
Hunter Handsfield, Richard P. DiCarlo, Adaora A. Adimora, Allen E. Izu,
Rhoda Ashley Morrow, and Lawrence Corey. "The Relationship between
Condom Use and Herpes Simplex Virus Acquisition." *Annals of Internal Medicine*
143, no. 10 (2005): 707–13.
Warner, Lee, Katherine M. Stone, Maurizio Macaluso, James W. Buehler, and
Harland D. Austin. "Condom Use and Risk of Gonorrhea and Chlamydia: A
Systematic Review of Design and Measurement Factors Assessed in
Epidemiologic Studies." *Sexually Transmitted Diseases* 33, no. 1 (2006): 36–51.

You Don't Need the HPV Vaccine If You're Not Having Sex

Alan Guttmacher Institute. "Sexual and Reproductive Health: Women and Men."
AGI, http://www.hawaii.edu/hivandaids/Sexual%20and%20Reproductive
%20Health%20%20%20%20Women%20and%20Men,%202002.pdf.
Chandra, Anjani, William D. Mosher, Casey Copen, and Catlainn Sionean. *Sexual
Behavior, Sexual Attraction, and Sexual Identity in the United States: Data from the
2006–2008 National Survey of Family Growth*: U.S. Department of Health and
Human Services, Centers for Disease Control and Prevention, National
Center for Health Statistics, 2011, 1–36.
Eaton, Danice K., Laura Kann, Steve Kinchen, Shari Shanklin, Katherine H. Flint,
Joseph Hawkins, William A. Harris, Richard Lowry, Tim McManus, and
David Chyen. "Youth Risk Behavior Surveillance—United States, 2011."
MMWR Surveillance Summaries 61, no. 4 (2012): 1–162.
Mosher, W. D., A. Chandra, and J. Jones. "Sexual Behavior and Selected Health

Measures: Men and Women 15–44 Years of Age, United States, 2002." *Advanced Data* 362 (2005): 1–55.

———. "Sexual Behavior and Selected Health Measures: Men and Women 15–44 Years of Age, United States, 2002." Mosher, W. D., Chandra, A., and J. Jones. *Advanced Data* 362 (2005): 1–55.

The HPV Vaccine Encourages Girls to Have Sex

Bednarczyk, Robert A., Robert Davis, Kevin Ault, Walter Orenstein, and Saad B. Omer. "Sexual Activity–Related Outcomes after Human Papillomavirus Vaccination of 11- to 12-Year-Olds." *Pediatrics* 130, no. 5 (2012): 798–805.

Eaton, D. K., L. Kann, S. Kinchen, S. Shanklin, J. Ross, J. Hawkins, W. A. Harris, R. Lowry, T. McManus, D. Chyen, C. Lim, L. Whittle, N. D. Brener, and H. Wechsler. "Youth Risk Behavior Surveillance—United States, 2009." *MMWR Morbidity and Mortality Weekly Report Surveillance Summaries* 59, no. 5 (2010): 1–142.

"Sexual Experience and Contraceptive Use among Female Teens—United States, 1995, 2002, and 2006–2010." *MMWR Morbidity and Mortality Weekly Report* 61, no. 17 (2012): 297–301.

You Better Not Kiss Anyone with HIV

Campo, J., M. A. Perea, J. del Romero, J. Cano, V. Hernando, and A. Bascones. "Oral Transmission of Hiv, Reality or Fiction? An Update." *Oral Diseases* 12, no. 3 (2006): 219–28.

Wahl, S. M., M. Redford, S. Christensen, W. Mack, J. Cohn, E. N. Janoff, J. Mestecky, H. B. Jenson, M. Navazesh, M. Cohen, P. Reichelderfer, and A. Kovacs. "Systemic and Mucosal Differences in Hiv Burden, Immune, and Therapeutic Responses." *Journal of Acquired Immune Deficiency Syndromes* 56, no. 5 (2011): 401–11.

Anal Sex Will Give You Cancer

Herbenick, Debby, Michael Reece, Vanessa Schick, Stephanie A. Sanders, Brian Dodge, and J. Dennis Fortenberry. "Sexual Behavior in the United States: Results from a National Probability Sample of Men and Women Ages 14–94." *Journal of Sexual Medicine* 7 (2010): 255–65.

Meyer, J. E., T. Narang, F. H. Schnoll-Sussman, M. B. Pochapin, P. J. Christos, and D. L. Sherr. "Increasing Incidence of Rectal Cancer in Patients Aged Younger Than 40 Years: An Analysis of the Surveillance, Epidemiology, and End Results Database." *Cancer* 116, no. 18 (2010): 4354–59.

Potterat, John J., Devon D. Brewer, and Stuart Brody. "Receptive Anal Intercourse as a Potential Risk Factor for Rectal Cancer." *Cancer* 117, no. 14 (2011): 3284–85.

Acknowledgments

We both need to thank the Indiana University School of Medicine Department of Pediatrics and the Division of Children's Health Services Research, as well as Riley Hospital for Children, for their support. We are incredibly grateful for our jobs, and both of us still marvel at the fact that we get paid to do things we love so much. We are also appreciative of our agents, Janet Rosen and Sheree Bykofsky, as well as our editor, Daniela Rapp, who inherited us, but treats us like we've been hers all along.

Aaron would additionally like to thank his family for their unending love and support. He would also like to acknowledge his friends, who often act like family, and know how to push his buttons. Although they couldn't contribute much to this book (thank goodness), life wouldn't be the same without his children—Jacob, Noah, and Sydney—for whom he is eternally grateful. But most of all, he wants to thank Aimee, whom he loves more each and every day. It's hard sometimes living with a person who thinks there's nothing you cannot do, but it's also the greatest gift he could have been given.

Rachel thanks her best friends for their constant love and support—Elizabeth Sparrow, Rebecca Vreeman Hoden, Maria Finnell, and Jessica Lasky Su. Life is better with sisters. She thanks Joe Fick, master baker, dog-father, and caretaker of all living things in his sphere. He has loved her well. Rachel also acknowledges and thanks her wonderful family, especially her always-supportive parents, Tom and Jacki Vreeman; her great brothers, Dan and Phil; and the nephews who are a constant source of smiles. She thanks Carole McAteer, who went above and beyond the call of research duty; and Michael Scanlon, who now shares her brain. Finally, Rachel thanks her travel buddies and the global health team of the I.U.–Kenya partnership, all of whom make her work and life adventures on both sides of the ocean so much more fun.

Index

abortions, IUD fears with, 192–93
acquired premature ejaculation, 142–43
adolescents. *See also* puberty
    premature ejaculation and, 141–43
    sex on television and, 134–35
affairs, 136–38
age. *See also* puberty
    anal sex frequency by, 140
    masturbation frequency by, 140
    oral sex frequency by, 140
    pornography consumption by, 145
    premature ejaculation and, 141–42
    pubic hair removal and, 82–83
    sperm changes with, 37–38
AIDS, 208. *See also* HIV
Akin, Todd, 183
alpha-adrenergic blockers, 47
American Academy of Family
        Physicians, 187
American Journal of Obstetrics & Gynecology,
    189–90
American Society for Microbiology, 208
anal sex
    age and frequency of, 140
    cancer and, 228–30
    cleanliness and, 108
    comfort with experimentation in,
        109–11
    condoms for, 157
    digital stimulation in, 98
    hemorrhoids and, 150–52
    HPV from, 229
    intravaginal intercourse combined
        with, 155–57
    men having orgasms with, 98
    penis size and, 11–13
    popularity of, 150, 155
    risks of, 107–10

sexually transmitted infections
        and, 229
    stigma of, 150
    women having orgasms from, 90,
        97–98
androstadienone, 160–61
antibiotics, birth control pill efficacy
        and, 187–88
anus
    bacteria inside, 156
    cleaning, 112–13
    sensitive regions of, 113
    stretching capability of, 108–10
aphrodisiacs, 101–5
Archives of Sexual Behavior, 137
artificial insemination, 181
athletic performance
    balance and, 30
    bras and, 55–56
    masturbation and, 28, 171
    sex impact on, 28–30

babies, gender manipulation and,
        197–99
bacterial vaginosis, 32, 156–57
"ball stretchers," 37
balls. *See* testicles
benign prostatic hyperplasia, 47
birth control. *See* condoms;
        intrauterine devices
birth control pills
    antibiotics and efficacy of, 187–88
    dosage calculation of, 189–90
    failure rates of, 187–91, 203
    obesity and efficacy of, 189–91
    side effects of, 186
    weight gain and, 185–86
blindness, masturbation and, 170–71

blond women
　　evolution and, 79–80
　　genetic origin of, 78
　　international popularity of, 77
　　male attraction to, 77
　　sex and, 80
boners. *See* erections
"bottoms," 12
brain
　　faked orgasms and, 167
　　G-spot and, 70
　　orgasms and women's, 91
　　sex impact on, 29–30
bras
　　athletic performance and, 55–56
　　comfort of, 56
　　sagging breasts and, 55–57
"Brazilian wax," 62, 65
breast cancer, 128
breasts
　　bras and sagging, 55–57
　　men's preferences with size of, 96
　　reconstructive surgery for, 95
　　size and sensitivity of, 94–96
　　squeezing, 127–28
　　stimulation of, 88, 90, 96, 127–28
　　studies on sensitivity of, 95–96
bush. *See* pubic hair

cadavers, orgasms and, 164–65
calories, sex burning, 119
cancer
　　anal sex and, 228–30
　　breast, 128
　　cervical, 212, 216, 229
　　colon, 228
cardiovascular disease, 172
cervical cancer, 212, 216, 229
cervix, 85, 179–80
cheating, 136–38
Chile, 131–32
China, 131
chlamydia, 207, 208, 212–13, 215

chocolate, as aphrodisiac, 101–4
chromosomes, 197–98
circumcision
　　benefits of, 32, 35
　　debate over, 31
　　disease prevention with, 32
　　global prevalence of, 31
　　HIV prevention with, 32
　　intravaginal intercourse duration
　　　　and, 26
　　orgasm and, 34
　　penis sensation and, 33–34
　　risks associated with, 33
　　studies on, 34–35
clamscaping, 62
cleanliness, sexually transmitted
　　　　infections and, 108, 112
clitoral orgasms, 10, 60
　　masturbation and, 89
　　vaginal orgasms compared to, 89–90
clitoris
　　function of, 60, 89
　　penis compared to, 72–73
　　piercing of, 122–23
　　stimulation of, 89–90
Clostridium difficile, 112
Cochrane Collaboration, 185–86
cocoa, 102–3
"Coital Alignment Technique," 11
coital incontinence, 74
cold sores, 213
colon cancer, 228
Columbia, 23
come. *See* ejaculate; semen
conception. *See* pregnancy
condoms, 178
　　for anal sex, 157
　　bacteria transmitted by, 156
　　breakage of, 162–63, 216–17
　　chlamydia protection with, 215
　　"double-bagging," 162–63
　　gonorrhea prevention with, 215
　　HIV prevention with, 216, 225

HSV protection with, 216
intravaginal intercourse duration and, 26
IUDs compared to, 194
men disliking, 163
oral sex and, 213
penis size problems with, 12
sexually transmitted infections and, 107
STD protection of, 215–17
Cooper's ligaments, 55
copper IUDs, 196
"core" housework, 116
cortisol, 160–61
crabs, 65–66, 210–11, 216
cum. *See* ejaculate; semen
Curculigo orchioides, 104

Dalkon Shield, 193–95
De Graaf, Reinjier, 73
dead people. *See* cadavers, orgasms and
Dead Serious News, 164
death, during sex, 172
decoagulation, sperm and, 180
"The Definitive Penis Size Survey," 20
Democratic Republic of Congo, 23
dental dam, 213
diabetes, 65
"double-bagging" condoms, 162–63
douching, 92–93, 157
Douglas, Michael, 212
dry orgasms, 46–47
dying pubic hair, 154

Ecuador, 23
education
infidelity and, 137
sex, 1
sex and level of, 131–32
eggs, 177–78, 185, 197–98, 200–203
Egypt, 93
ejaculate. *See also* semen
swallowing, 44–45
volume of, 39–41

ejaculation. *See also* squirting
of cadavers, 164–65
duration before, 25–27
of men compared to squirting of women, 72–73
nocturnal, 168–69
orgasms in men without, 46–47
"point of no return" and, 47
premature, 11, 25–27
sperm quantity per, 50–51, 198
in water, 202–3
women and, 70
electrolysis, 63, 82
embarrassment
broken penis and, 49
premature ejaculation and, 27
wet dreams and, 168–69
emissions. *See* ejaculation
erectile dysfunction, 172
erections. *See also* penis
breaking, 48–49
cadavers and, 165
penis size and, 14, 16
penis size from flaccid to, 42–43
priapism and, 165
estrogen, 139, 185
ethnicity
douching by, 92
penis size and, 22–24
pubic hair grooming and, 83–84
evolution
blond women and, 79–80
penis size and, 8–9, 23–24
pregnancy and, 183
sexual selection and, 78–80
exercise, sex as, 119–20
experimenting, with sex, 106–13

faking orgasms, women, 166–67
fellatio, 226. *See also* oral sex
female ejaculation. *See* squirting
female orgasmic disorder, 60
female sexual arousal disorder, 60

fertility, IUDs impacting, 194–96
flaccid penis size, 16, 42–43
flavonoids, 103
food, aphrodisiacs and, 101–5
foot size, penis size and, 18–21
foreskin, 31–35. *See also* circumcision
Framingham Heart Study, 172–73
France, 196

gender manipulation, pregnancy and,
   197–99
genetics, 197–98
genital ulcers, 216
genital warts, 212, 216, 222–23
  penis size and, 12
germs, from toilet seats, 207–9
Ghana, 23
gonorrhea, 107, 207, 208, 212–13
  condoms preventing, 215
Gräfenberg, Ernst, 67–68, 73, 76
graying, of pubic hair, 153–54
group sex, comfort and, 109–10
G-spot
  arguments against, 69–70
  arguments for, 70–71
  brain and, 70
  debate over, 67
  definition of, 67
  discovery of, 67–68, 73
  nerve endings in, 68–69
  science and existence of, 69
  women's belief in, 68
The G-Spot: And Other Recent Discoveries
   About Human Sexuality (Perry and
   Whipple), 68
Guttmacher Institute, 218

hair color, 77–80, 153–54. *See also* blond
   women; pubic hair
hand size, penis size and, 18–21
happiness
  infidelity and, 138
  wealth and, 132–33

health research
  scrutiny of, 3
  for sex myths, 2
  sexual frequency and, 124–26
heart attacks, sex and, 172–74
height, penis size and, 9
hematoma, 33
hemoglobin, 196
hemorrhoids
  anal sex and, 150–52
  causes of, 151
  common occurrence of, 150
  internal, 150
  treating, 151
herbs, as aphrodisiac, 102, 104–5
herpes, 64, 107, 207, 208, 212–13
  penis size and, 12
herpes simplex virus (HSV), 216
HIV, 107, 207. *See also* AIDS
  circumcision preventing, 32
  condoms preventing, 216, 225
  international prevalence of, 224
  kissing and, 224–27
  medication treating, 224
  from oral sex, 213, 225–27
  in pregnancy, 225
  spreading, 157
  transmission of, 224–25
housework, sex and sharing,
   114–16
Hox gene, 18–19
HPV. *See* human papillomavirus
HSV. *See* herpes simplex virus
human life span, sex and, 124–26
human papillomavirus (HPV), 107,
   212, 216
  from anal sex, 229
  intravaginal intercourse and, 229
  vaccine for, 218–20
hypoactive sexual desire disorder, 60

India, 135, 162
infertility, IUDs and, 194–96

infidelity, men and, 136–38
insertion, sex and, 106–13
internal hemorrhoids, 150
Internet
    cadavers and orgasms on, 164
    penis size survey on, 7–8,
      15, 22
    pornography on, 144
intrauterine devices (IUDs)
    abortion fears with, 192–93
    bleeding or pain with, 196
    condoms compared to, 194
    copper, 196
    effectiveness of, 192
    fertility impact of, 194–96
    infections from, 193–94
    popularity of, 192
intravaginal intercourse
    anal sex combined with, 155–57
    average duration of, 26, 119
    circumcision and duration of, 26
    condoms and duration of, 26
    HPV and, 229
    measuring duration of, 27
    premature ejaculation and, 25
    "pulling out" and, 200–201
IQ, racial stereotypes and, 24
Italy, 135
IUDs. *See* intrauterine devices

*JAMA. See The Journal of the American
    Medical Association*
Japan, 56
Johnson, Virginia E., 42
Journal of Sex Research, 168
*The Journal of the American Medical
    Association (JAMA),* 141–42

Kama Sutra, 73, 121
Kenya, 34, 77
Kinsey, Alfred, 168
Kinsey Institute, 15, 43, 91, 139
kissing, HIV and, 224–27

laser hair removal, 63, 81–82
latex sheet, 213
laundry, marital satisfaction
    and, 114–16
Litsea chinensis, 104
lubricant, 113
Lynn, Richard, 23–24

marijuana, 104
marriage, 58–60
    infidelity and, 136–38
    masturbation and, 158–59
    sex and satisfaction with, 114–16
    sexual desire and, 148
    "trophy wives" and, 136
    wealth and, 130–33
Masters, William H., 42
masturbation
    age and frequency of, 140
    athletic performance and, 28, 171
    benefits of, 171
    blindness and, 170–71
    clitoral orgasms and, 89
    marriage and, 158–59
    men's frequency compared to
      women's, 158
    popularity of, 170
    sex myths and fears with, 170
    sperm depletion from, 51
    vaginal orgasms and, 89
McGlone, S., 28–29
men. *See also* penis; penis size
    anal sex orgasms of, 98
    blond women's attractiveness
      to, 77
    breast size preferences of, 96
    condoms disliked by, 163
    HPV vaccine for, 222–23
    infidelity and, 136–38
    orgasms without ejaculation
      in, 46–47
    penis size in men having sex
      with, 11–13

men. *(continued)*
    penis size satisfaction of, 7–8, 12
    piercing of, 121–23
    pornography habits of women
        compared to, 144–46
    public hair removal and, 64, 84
    sexual peak of women compared to,
        139–40
    squirting of women compared to
        ejaculation of, 72–73
    sweat and, 160–61
    wet dreams and, 168–69
    women enjoying housework
        performed by, 114–16
    women's frequency of masturbation
        compared to, 158
    women's sexual arousal compared
        to, 59
    women's sexual desire compared to,
        147–49
meningitis, 188
menstrual cycle, 177–78
mites, 210
molluscum contagiosum, 64
money. *See* wealth
monogamy, women and, 58–60
mons pubis, 62
multiple orgasms, of women, 60
multiple partners, 109–10
myths. *See* sex myths

the Netherlands, 77, 117–18
Nettle, Daniel, 130
The New England Journal of Medicine,
    194–95
New Zealand, 122, 195
nipples, stimulating, 127–28.
    See also breasts
nitric oxide, 103
nocturnal emissions, 168–69
Norway, 195
nose size, penis size and, 20
nude sleep, 129

obesity, birth control pills efficacy
    and, 189–91
ointments, 194
oral cavity, 227
oral herpes, 213
oral sex
    age and frequency of, 140
    condoms and, 213
    HIV from, 213, 225–27
    pregnancy and, 212
    pubic hair and, 62, 83
    safety of, 212–14
    STDs from, 212–14
    vaginal orgasms and, 98
orgasms. *See also* ejaculation
    cadavers and, 164–65
    circumcision and, 34
    clitoral, 10, 60, 89–90
    "Coital Alignment Technique"
        and, 11
    dry, 46–47
    historical debates on, 72
    men having anal sex, 98
    of men without ejaculation, 46–47
    penis size and women's, 10–11
    piercings and, 123
    pregnancy and, 179–82
    sock removal and, 117–18
    spinal cord injuries and, 88–89
    spontaneous, 88
    vaginal, 10, 89–90, 98
    wealth and, 131–32
    women and multiple, 60
    women faking, 166–67
    women having anal sex,
        90, 97–98
    women's brain and, 91
    women's challenges with, 91
    women's mechanisms for, 88
    zone, 88
ovulation, 177
oxytocin, 181
oysters, as aphrodisiac, 101–2

pajamas, sleep habits and, 129
pelvic infection, 194, 195–96
"penile manipulation," 48
penis. *See also* erections
     bacteria transmitted by, 156
     breaking, 48–49
     circumcision and sensation of, 33–34
     clitoris compared to, 72–73
     after death, 164–65
     flexibility of, 48
     growth of, 42–43
     piercing of, 121–23
     priapism and, 165
penis size
     anal sex and, 11–13
     attraction and, 9
     average, 15–17, 43
     condom problems with, 12
     discussions over, 14
     erections and, 14, 16
     ethnicity and, 22–24
     evolution and, 8–9, 23–24
     flaccid, 16, 42–43
     from flaccid to erection, 42–43
     foot size and, 18–21
     genital warts and herpes and, 12
     hand size and, 18–21
     height and, 9
     Internet survey on, 7–8, 15, 22
     measuring, 14–17, 19, 22
     in men having sex with men, 11–13
     men satisfaction with, 7–8, 12
     nose size and, 20
     physical traits associate with large, 8
     popular opinion on, 7–8
     racial stereotypes and, 22–24
     self satisfaction with, 8, 13
     shoe size and, 19–20
     studies on, 15–17, 19–20, 22–23
     techniques for studying, 16, 19, 22
     vaginal orgasms and, 10
     women satisfaction with, 8–10
     women's orgasms and, 10–11

period, 177–78
periurethral glands, 73
Perry, John, 68
persistent genital arousal disorder, 61
petroleum jelly, 113
phenylethylamine, 104
piercings, 121–23
the pill. *See* birth control pills
Pioneer Fund, 24
plants, as aphrodisiac, 104–5
Playboy, 77, 82
"point of no return," ejaculation and, 47
politics, rape and, 183
Pollet, Thomas, 130
pornography
     age and consumption of, 145
     habits of men compared to
          women, 144–46
     on Internet, 144
     profitability of, 145
     pubic hair and, 63
     squirting in, 75
     stereotypes with, 144
     women's response to, 58–59
posterior urethral valves, 46–47
pregnancy. *See also* birth control pills;
          condoms; intrauterine devices
     artificial insemination and, 181
     bacterial vaginosis and, 156
     douching impact on, 93
     evolution and, 183
     gender manipulation and, 197–99
     HIV in, 225
     HPV vaccine and, 221–22
     menstrual cycle and, 177–78
     oral sex and, 212
     orgasms and, 179–82
     "pulling out" and, 200–201
     rape and, 183–84
     rhythm method and, 178
     sex in water and, 202–3
     sex myths with, 200–203
     sex standing up to avoid, 201–2

pregnancy *(continued)*
　sexual caution with, 110
　sperm and, 45, 51–52
premature ejaculation, 11, 25–27
　acquired, 142–43
　adolescents and, 141–43
　age and, 141–42
　definition and guidelines of, 25
　diagnosing, 25
　embarrassment and, 27
　intravaginal intercourse and, 25
　lifelong, 142
　media perception of, 143
　solution for, 27
　studies on, 25–26
priapism, 165
Prince Albert piercing, 121
progestin, 185
progestogen, 192
prolapsed uterus, 179
prostate gland, 72
puberty. *See also* adolescents
　pubic hair and, 81
　testicles and, 36
pubic hair
　age and removal of, 82–83
　crabs and, 210–11, 216
　dying, 154
　ethnicity and grooming of, 83–84
　function of, 64
　graying of, 153–54
　income level and grooming of, 83
　men removing, 64, 84
　oral sex and, 62, 83
　pornography and, 63
　puberty and, 81
　public pressure on grooming, 82
　reasons for removing, 62–63
　risks and injuries in removal of,
　　63–65
　trends in, 81–84
　viruses and infections with removal
　　of, 64–65
　vulva protected by, 64
　women's grooming of, 62–66, 81–84
pubic lice, 65–66, 210–11, 216
"pulling out," pregnancy and,
　200–201

racial stereotypes. *See also* ethnicity
　IQ and, 24
　penis size and, 22–24
rape, 110
　politics and, 183
　pregnancy and, 183–84
rectum. *See also* anal sex
　bacteria inside, 156
　cleaning, 112–13
　stretching capability of, 108–10
redheads, 77–80
religion, infidelity and, 137
rhythm method, pregnancy and, 178
rifampin, 188
Rouillon, Jean-Denis, 56–57
Rushton, J. Philippe, 23–24

saliva, 227
scabies, 210–11
scrotum, 36, 37
SEER. *See* Surveillance, Epidemiology,
　　and End Results
semen. *See also* ejaculate; sperm
　cleanliness of, 44
　production of, 72
　"running out" of, 50–52
　swallowing, 44–45
　volume of, 39–41
seminal vesicles, 72
"seven-year itch," 136
sex. *See also* anal sex
　accurate information on, 1
　aphrodisiacs and, 101–5
　athletic performance and, 28–30
　blond women and, 80
　body part combinations tried in, 106–7
　brain impact of, 29–30

calories burned in, 119
cleanliness and, 108
comfort with experimentation
    in, 109–11
death during, 172
duration of, 25–27, 119
education, 1
education level and, 131–32
energy used during, 29
as exercise, 119–20
exhaustion from, 29
experimenting with, 106–13
group, 109–10
health research on frequency
    of, 124–26
heart attacks and, 172–74
housework sharing and, 114–16
human life span and, 124–26
insertion and, 106–13
marital satisfaction and, 114–16
marriage and desire for, 148
men's desire compared to women's
    with, 147–49
physical exertion of, 173–74
pregnancy and standing up for, 201–2
pregnancy caution with, 110
"pulling out" and, 200–201
risks of experimental, 107–10, 155
sleep habits and, 129
sock removal for, 117–18
television and, 134–35
in water, 202–3
wealth and, 130–33
women's desire for, 58–61, 116
sex myths. *See also specific myths*
    busting, 1–3
    data for addressing, 2–3
    health research for, 2
    masturbation fears and, 170
    with pregnancy, 200–203
sex of baby, manipulating, 197–99
sexual arousal
    female sexual arousal disorder and, 60
    of men compared to women, 59
    persistent genital arousal disorder
        and, 61
    smell and, 160
    sweat and, 160–61
sexual assault, 110
sexual peak, 139–40
sexual selection, 78–80
sexually transmitted diseases (STDs)
    condom protection from, 215–17
    from oral sex, 212–14
    toilet seats and, 207–9
sexually transmitted infections
    anal sex and, 229
    bacterial vaginosis increasing risk of,
        156
    bleeding and tearing increasing risk
        of, 107–8
    cleanliness preventing, 108, 112
    condoms and, 107
    crabs, 65–66, 210–11
    objects carrying, 112
    protection from, 155
    scabies, 210–11
    transmission of, 107
shaving, 63, 82
shoe size, penis size and, 19–20
Shrier, I., 28–29
sleep habits
    sex and, 129
    television and, 135
smell
    sexual arousal and, 160
    sweat and, 160–61
    of vagina, 86–87
sock removal, for sex, 117–18
sperm, 200. *See also* semen
    age changes with, 37–38
    decoagulation and, 180
    genetics in, 197–98
    gravity and, 201–2
    life span of, 177–78
    masturbation depleting, 51

sperm *(continued)*
  per ejaculation, 50–51, 198
  pregnancy and, 45, 51–52
  production of, 50–52, 72
  speed of, 198
  "upsuck" and, 179, 181
  vaginal travel of, 180
spermicides, 196
sphincter, stretching of, 109
spinal cord injuries, orgasms and, 88–89
spontaneous orgasms, 88
squirting. *See also* ejaculation
  ejaculation of men compared to
    women and, 72–73
  historical accounts of, 73
  in pornography, 75
  studies on, 74–76
  urethra and, 73
  urine in, 73–76
STDs. *See* sexually transmitted diseases
Stewart, Martha, 212
Streptococcus pyogenes, 65
Surveillance, Epidemiology, and End
    Results (SEER), 228–29
sweat, sexual arousal and, 160–61

tampons, lost in vagina, 85–87
teenagers. *See* adolescents; puberty
television, sex and, 134–35
testicles
  hanging of, 36–37
  puberty and, 36
  sagging of, 36–38
  stretching, 37
testosterone, peak levels of, 139
Thailand, 163
toilet seats
  crabs and scabies from, 210–11
  STDs and, 207–9
"tops," 13
toxic shock syndrome, 86
Trichomonas, 32
"trophy wives," 136

tuberculosis, 188
Turkey, 26, 93

United States, 62, 63, 83, 124, 129, 132,
    141, 144, 170, 184, 193, 219, 221
"upsuck," 179, 181
urethra, 73, 106
urine
  coital incontinence and, 74
  squirting and, 73–76
  stopping flow of, 47
  on toilet seats, 208
uterus, 179, 181–82, 192. *See also*
    intrauterine devices

vaccine, HPV, 221–23
vagina
  bacteria inside, 155–57
  bacterial vaginosis and, 32, 156
  cleaning, 112–13
  discharging objects from, 87
  douching for cleaning, 92–93, 157
  G-spot, 67–71
  "pulling out" of, 200–201
  sensitive regions of, 113
  smell of, 86–87
  sperm travel within, 180
  stretching capability of, 86, 108–10
  tampons and objects lost in, 85–87
  tearing of, 110
  toxic shock syndrome and, 86
vaginal orgasms
  clitoral orgasms compared to, 89–90
  masturbation and, 89
  oral sex and, 98
  penis size and, 10
"vaginal tenting," 180–81
vajazzling, 62
vibrators, 74, 170
vulva, pubic hair protecting, 64

water, sex in, 202–3
waxing, 62–65, 81–82

wealth
  happiness and, 132–33
  infidelity and, 137
  marriage and sex impact of, 130–33
  orgasms and, 131–32
  self-esteem and, 131
weight gain, birth control pill and,
    185–86
wet dreams, 168–69
Whipple, Beverly, 68
women. *See also* breasts; clitoral
    orgasms; clitoris; pregnancy;
    vagina
  anal sex orgasms of, 90, 97–98
  blond, 77–80
  bras and sagging breasts of, 55–57
  breast size and sensitivity of, 94–96
  ejaculation and, 70
  ejaculation of men compared to
    squirting of, 72–73
  G-spot belief of, 68
  HPV vaccine and, 221–23
  men performing housework for,
    114–16
  men's frequency of masturbation
    compared to, 158
  men's sexual arousal compared to, 59

  men's sexual desire compared
    to, 147–49
  monogamy and, 58–60
  multiple orgasms of, 60
  orgasm challenges of, 91
  orgasm mechanisms of, 88
  orgasms and brain of, 91
  orgasms faked by, 166–67
  penis size and orgasms of, 10–11
  penis size satisfaction of, 8–10
  piercing of, 121–23
  pornography habits of men
    compared to, 144–46
  pornography response of, 58–59
  pubic hair grooming of, 62–66, 81–84
  sexual desire of, 58–61, 116
  sexual peak of men compared
    to, 139–40
  sweat and, 160–61
  wet dreams and, 168–69

X chromosomes, 197–98

Y chromosomes, 197–98
yeast infections, 156

zone orgasms, 88

About the Authors

Photograph by Eric Lubrick

Aaron E. Carroll, MD, MS, is a professor of pediatrics, Assistant Dean for Research Mentoring, and Director of the Center for Health Policy and Professionalism Research at the Indiana University School of Medicine. He has earned a BA in Chemistry from Amherst College, an MD from the University of Pennsylvania School of Medicine, and a master's degree in Health Services from the University of Washington. He loves to read, ski, watch TV, collect comic books, play video games, write, talk on the radio, eat good food, drink good alcohol, and play with his kids. He blogs regularly at The Incidental Economist (http://theincidentalconomist.com) and is a contributor to CNN.com on health and health policy. He lives with his wife and three children in Carmel, Indiana.

Photograph by Eric Lubrick

Rachel C. Vreeman, MD, MS, is an assistant professor of pediatrics at the Indiana University School of Medicine and Co-Director of Pediatric Research for the Academic Model Providing Access to Healthcare (AMPATH) in Kenya. She has earned a BA in English from Cornell University, an MD from the Michigan State University College of Human Medicine, and a master's degree in Clinical Research from Indiana University. Rachel lives out of a suitcase on two continents and blogs about her global health work and travels at

Doctor V Goes Over the Sea (http://doctorvoversea.com). She will eat anything (except potatoes) and go anywhere. Rachel loves new adventures, devouring books, taking photographs, her puppies, a glass of wine, and—most of all—laughing with the people she loves.

Aaron and Rachel are the coauthors of *Don't Swallow Your Gum! Myths, Half-Truths, and Outright Lies About Your Body and Health* and *Don't Cross Your Eyes . . . They'll Get Stuck That Way! And 75 Other Health Myths Debunked.*